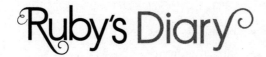

Ruby's Diary

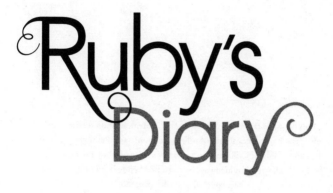

Ruby's Diary

Reflections on All I've
Lost and Gained

Ruby Gettinger
with Sheryl Berk

WM

WILLIAM MORROW

An Imprint of HarperCollins*Publishers*

B GETTINGER

RUBY'S DIARY. Copyright © 2009 by E! Entertainment Television Inc. All rights reserved. Printed in the United States of America. No part of this book may be used or reproduced in any manner whatsoever without written permission except in the case of brief quotations embodied in critical articles and reviews. For information address HarperCollins Publishers, 10 East 53rd Street, New York, NY 10022.

HarperCollins books may be purchased for educational, business, or sales promotional use. For information please write: Special Markets Department, HarperCollins Publishers, 10 East 53rd Street, New York, NY 10022.

FIRST EDITION

Designed by Jamie Lynn Kerner

Library of Congress Cataloging-in-Publication Data has been applied for.

ISBN 978-0-06-192460-6

09 10 11 12 13   OV/RRD   10 9 8 7 6 5 4 3 2 1

For everyone who suffers from an addiction;
everyone who has had something take control
over them and has wondered where
that something came from;
everyone who asks themselves
that frightening question
"Can I ever conquer this thing?"
and continues to believe that
they can despite the odds,
I stand up and applaud each of you;
you are my heroes.

—R. G.

CONTENTS

Acknowledgments xiii

Dear Friends 1

CHAPTER ONE: GETTING STARTED 7

You Never Know What God's Gonna Do 7

Here She Goes Again . . . 10

The End . . . Almost 11

New Beginnings 14

CHAPTER TWO: UPS AND DOWNS 17

Fighting the Beast 17

"I Love That Song!" 18

A Shout-Out to BIG Fans Everywhere:

 A Letter to Miley Cyrus 20

Love Letters 21

From the Hearts of Brittany Daniel and

 Cynthia Daniel Hauser 22

CHAPTER THREE: CRAVINGS 25

Medium-Size Wish List 25

Extra-Large Wish List

 (Newly Expanded to Include More Fun!) 26

Hunger Pains 30

Pizza Envy   31
My Ten Most Wanted Foods   33
New and Improved Favorites   35
From the Heart of Danna Kirk   36

CHAPTER FOUR:
SOUTHERN HOSPITALITY AND CHARM   38
Savory Savannah   38
Georgia on My Mind   41
Another Ax to Grind   43
Just One Slice   43
Am I Supposed to Eat This?   45
A Note from Ruby's Physician   47
Tips from Ruby's Diet Doctor   49
From Dietician Kate Melei:
    The Cost-Conscious Seven-Day Meal Plan   51

CHAPTER FIVE: MISSING MORE THAN FOOD   55
Why Can't I Remember?   55
You-Know-Who Keeps Callin' Me!   57
Where'd All the Romance Go?   58
There's a Comfort in Being Fat   63
From the Heart of Marcia Thompson   64

CHAPTER SIX: A CHANGE IS GONNA COME   67
Back to Work   67
The Christmas Doctor   71
Bribing Georgia   71

Testing Positive for Strength   72
From the Heart of Georgia Thompson   74

CHAPTER SEVEN: MY HEAVY HEART   76
I Miss My Daddy So Much   76
Denny to the Rescue   82
Back in the Groove   83
Another Family Crisis   85
My Angel Boy   86
From the Heart of Denny Starr   87
Ruby's Smile   89

CHAPTER EIGHT: TIRED OF WEIGHTING   92
L.A. or Bust   92
Where Did I Go Wrong?   93
Reading the Writing on the Label   94
Birthday Party Blues   95
From the Heart of Jim Gettinger   98

CHAPTER NINE: MAKING WAVES   100
Best Lifeguards Ever   100
The Big Fight   101
Truce   103
Finally Out of the Fours   104
From the Heart of Georgia's Sons,
     Ben and Zach Thompson   105

CONTENTS

CHAPTER TEN: FREEDOM   107

Baby, I Can Drive My Car!   107

Road Rage   108

Just Say No   109

The Finish Line   110

From the Heart of Jeff Parsons   111

CHAPTER ELEVEN: EXTRA SUPPORT   114

That Don't Come in My Size   114

Me on the Runway   117

Keepin' the Faith   118

This Could Have Been Me   120

Living My Best Life: A Letter to Oprah Winfrey   122

Now I'm Cookin'!   124

From the Heart of Julie Gannam   127

CHAPTER TWELVE: LET'S GET PHYSICAL   129

The Start of Something New   129

Row, Row, Row Your Boat   132

Having a Ball   136

I Like to Move It, Move It . . .   137

My Current Workout   140

A Note from Ruby's Trainers   141

CHAPTER THIRTEEN:
CHILDHOOD HOPES AND DREAMS   143

The Two Faces of Ruby Gettinger   143

A Dark and Stormy Night   144

Picture This   145

The Music Man   147

Uggy People   148

Baby Talk   150

From the Heart of Leslie McGinty   154

CHAPTER FOURTEEN: ALMOST FAMOUS   156

R-E-S-P-E-C-T   156

A Little More Than a Dozen Eyes on Me   158

Rosie Thoughts   159

That's an Easy Question . . .   160

Rubyisms   161

Be the Change: A Letter to President Obama   163

From the Heart of Christine Acosta   165

CHAPTER FIFTEEN: FINAL WORDS   167

Opening a New Door   167

If God Could Change Anything . . .   168

Ruby's Resource Guide   171

ACKNOWLEDGMENTS

I wish to thank my family and friends: Daddy (my hero), Mom (the light of my life), Clyde, Brenda, Jim Gettinger, Steve, Jamie, Karen White, John Gettinger, Georgia, Ben, Zach Thompson, Jeff Parsons, Foxy, Lucy, Mellie, Leslie and Greg McGinty, Marcia Thompson, Danna Kirk, Chris Acosta, Toni Suchka, Brittany Daniel, Denny Starr, Cynthia and Cole Hauser, David King, Dr. Ahmed, Anna, Katcha, Irina Tuytina, Tomas Aguiar, Michael and Melissa Leland, Judy Thomas, Julie Gunnam, Tonya Mounkes, Chellie Heckman, Vernita Washington, Judy Kemp, Joan White, Maxine Sussman.

My Prayer Warriors: my aunt Georgette, Greg, Leslie, Gary, Miles, Matthew, Grace, Graham, Maryanna McGinty, Marcia Thompson, Barbara Parsons, Ann Moore, Irma Collins, John and Barbra McGinty, Paul Alexander, Sue Davis, and the Sanctuary and CBC of Savannah.

Brittany Daniel for caring enough about my journey to approach Tim Puntillo. Gratitude to you both from the bottom of my heart for getting my story out there! Thank you, too, Amy Daneles for helping us get the first pilot shot!

Special thanks to The Style Network for believing in me and caring enough about this addiction to help me make a change. Ted Harbert, you have my heartfelt appreciation for taking a chance with me; Suzanne Kolb, I value your friendship and loyalty; Salaam Coleman Smith, I am thankful to you for your heart and for telling my truth; Sarah Weidman and Elaine Brooks, warm thanks to you for keeping my vision alive; Carrie Franklin, your faith and belief in me is amazing; Melissa Stone, thank you for your devotion; Lisa Working, thank you for working so hard; Grace Borrero, thank you for your ongoing support; Domenic Morea, thank you for your faith and drive and for never giving up. Janelle Albino, Leigh Anne Gardner, and everyone else I have met face-to-face or talked to on the phone, you all have my heartfelt appreciation, too! And to Gay Rosenthal Productions: what an amazing journey we've taken together! Thank you to each and every one of you who helped make it all possible, whether you were here for a short while or along for the full ride: Gay Rosenthal, Nicholas Caprio, Paul Barosse, Victoria Zielinski, Harry Frith, Myrna Everett, Tara Higgins, Charlise Holmes, Whitney Ince, Eric Streit, Ally Hilliard, Jason Vernon, Dustin Everett, and anyone else I may have missed, I am so happy to have made so many friends for life!

Thank you to my original team of experts for setting me off in the right direction: Dr. Steven Course, Dr. Paul Bradley, Mindy Bradley, Helen Hussey, Reese Brown, and Dr. Tim Brewerton. I will always be grateful. Thank you also to the folks at Hourglass/Ourlife. Dr. Bradley, I'm especially grateful that you are making it affordable for all people to address diabetes and obesity in America. Thank you for sharing my vision. Drew and Shazia Edmonds, my new trainers, who have

ACKNOWLEDGMENTS

motivated me and helped me reach the goals I have set for myself. You are my soul mate trainers!

Thank you to the families that have sacrificed while their loved ones are away shooting my journey. Thank you to the wonderful city of Savannah, Georgia. Your beauty and southern charm make you a character all on your own! Thank you, Frank Stewart, Paula Bolden, and Iris Grossman for your friendship and good counsel!

Thank you to all the Ruby ambassadors, especially Rob Dempsey, who constantly promotes my show on radio because he, too, wants people to beat the Beast no matter what their Beast may be, and to all who cheer me on via letters, e-mail, MySpace, Twitter, Facebook, and more.

Thank you to the publishing team that helped develop and market this book— Suzanne Kolb, Stephen Earley, David Palmer, John Wilson, Robert Carrasco, Mark Scheider, and Angelo Lopipero at Comcast; Hope Innelli, Liate Stehlik, Lynn Grady, Seale Ballenger, Jean Marie Kelly, Brianne Halverson, Shawn Nicholls, Tom Ward, Beth Silfin, Judy DeGrottole, and Richard Aquan at HarperCollins; and Sheryl Berk— for all their dedication, hard work, and patience. Sheryl, you are an angel and I thank you, my new friend!

Thank You to God for never giving up on me, and for giving me the purpose and destiny I feel You have put before me. I pray I make You and everyone on this mission with me proud. To everyone who supported and believed in me as I crossed your paths, I have been inspired by you and am a better person for our meeting.

Lastly, I want to acknowledge four precious people in memory: my sweet Jeanie Gill, Morgan Parsons, and Caleb Parsons, who were all taken from this life too early, you inspired and touched many! And to James Gettinger, who lost his battle with diabetes, my love for you lives on. Prayers and love to all.

ACKNOWLEDGMENTS

Ruby's Diary

Dear Friends:

I know that "hey, y'all" is the typical southern greeting. But if you are buying this book or just browsing through it at the bookstore, then I'm pretty sure you or someone you know is dealing with weight issues just like me, and in that case, y'all are my friends. Lately I'm just shocked at how big this inner circle of mine has gotten.

I used to think that when I grew up I would be a psychiatrist. I wanted to help people solve their problems. But if someone had told me, "Ruby, you're gonna be on a television show someday and the whole world is gonna watch you struggle with your problems," I would have just laughed and said, "Are you crazy? There is no way under the sun, moon, and stars I would ever let someone follow me around and put my body on national TV! That would scare even the bears out of the forest!" And I would have thought they were even crazier if they told me I was gonna write a book. No, this is not at all what I had in mind, I swear. Not that I'm complaining, because I believe it is a great gift I have been given. Even when it seems like a sacrifice. Even when it's all hangin' out there for everyone to see: the good, the bad, the "oh no, where did those five extra, freakin' pounds come from?!"

I guess because it did all seem so unexpected, I just knew that it was out of my hands; it was destiny that I do this. That's why I have this little pet name for my journal: I call her "Destiny," 'cause that's what I'm living now—my destiny.

I know a diary is supposed to be something no one else sees; something you hide away under lock and key. But anyone who's ever met me knows that I am all about being open and honest and telling the truth, the whole truth, and nothin' but the truth. So while I was writing down all of these thoughts of mine, I realized that there were still so many more things that I wanted to share with my friends, my supporters watching the show, and my team of experts. That's when I decided to put some entries in a special book for y'all to read. A few of them cover issues I needed to revisit for myself, but most go beyond what you see on the show or read on my Web site. I didn't include everything, of course. The book would be longer than Gone With the Wind if I did! I just chose the entries that are my favorites. Some made me laugh; others made me cry; a few even terrified me. But they're all important because they're a part of me. They're my story, which I am continuing to discover piece by piece, page by page.

As many of you know—and some of you are about to find out—my story doesn't have a beginning yet because I can't remember a lot of my past. And I certainly don't know how it's all gonna end. But I am hoping that paying attention to the stuff in the middle—the stuff I'm going through right now—the rest of my story will fall into place. It's like I'm working on a great big puzzle and I lost some of the pieces. Everything I do, every corner I turn, could help me find one of those pieces. Even writing this book can help me do that.

Unlike the show, my diary is a little "raw"—I like to think of it as "Ruby Unplugged"! Sometimes I can get very deep. Like when I sit here wondering, "What's my life about? How did I get here? Where am I going? What is my passion? And how am I gonna pursue it?" Other times, I write about how I'm feeling at the moment: "Today's been a hard day for me; I've had a severe, severe headache. I've had the shakes; I'm still having the shakes. I think I am having sugar withdrawal . . ."

Then there's the mean and ornery entries. They represent "The Dark Side of Ruby," as I like to call it, the times when I'm frustrated. The times when I just gotta let my thoughts out so they don't boil up inside me. The times when I'm good and mad and just wanna tell someone about it. That's when I write things like: "I feel so agitated, my jaw is tight. And that's because right now I'm just not a 'hacky' camper because I feel like I'm starving. I wake up starving and I go to sleep starving. I am hungry 24/7! I know this food they gave me is good for me, but I just don't like it and it don't fill me up! I freakin' miss my spaghetti!" Fortunately for y'all, there are more fun and thoughtful entries than ornery ones, but if I spared you the truth about the tough days, I'd be lying to you.

I also like to write letters in my diary. Until now, I wasn't sure I would ever show some of these to anyone. In them, I tell people what I really think they oughta know. I express what's truly in my heart. They are a way for me to share words that I don't say face-to-face to people even though they are near and dear to me, and I should. Sometimes they are a way for me to say what I was thinking, but didn't dare mention at the time because I'm way too much of a lady to go there. (Isn't that what diaries are for, y'all!? Blowin' off steam!) And finally, some of these letters are a way for me to say the things I wish I could just shout out from a mountaintop or advertise on a big old billboard so the whole world would wake up and take notice.

On the TV show, you see me struggling and whining; sweating and panting; winning and losing. Sometimes I'm not really sure what y'all must be thinking, but most times I'm hoping that you are learning something about yourself while you're watching me. It's the same with this book. I'm hoping that reading it will help us all learn something.

I can't say it often enough: we are a nation in the middle of an obesity epidemic, and I am determined to find out why. I don't mind being the "guinea pig" if it means we'll all finally get some answers, because there are a lot of lies out there about this disease. There are the lies that other people spread about it and about the people who have it, and there are the lies those of us suffering from it tell ourselves. But I know the truth. I confront it every day. And I'm doing all I can to share that truth with the world.

When I started dieting at age eight, I never knew how hard life was going to be. By the time I invited cameras into my life, I understood that I would be vulnerable and I would be exposing my private feelings and emotions to the world. But what I never knew was how mental this would all be! Even after wrapping our second season, I'm still on an emotional ride! I'm still finding out new things about myself I never could have imagined. I'm still seeing myself in a way that I hadn't ever looked at myself before. Each one of the episodes on TV is only thirty minutes, and that's not an awful lot of time for people to see everything that's really going on with me. There is so much more! And that's where my diary and this book fit in. They let me explain a lot to myself and to you.

This is where I get to say things I didn't have a chance to say before, or maybe where I get to confront feelings I was afraid to even let myself have. This is where I get to tell people how much they mean to me, and I get to let loose and just be me, Ruby.

It is hard work, but you know, it didn't take long for me to find comfort and purpose in it. I am really blessed to have people around me every day who believe in me and who support my vision. Everyone—my friends, my family, my team of experts, the producers, my director of photography, the crew, and you—all help me realize that this journey has been worth the risk of putting myself out there. So now, in a way, I'm turning over the key to my diary. You can read it whenever or wherever you like. May it help you as much as it is helping me.

Hugs and well-wishes,

Ruby

1 GETTING STARTED

You Never Know What God's Gonna Do

I was on the treadmill today thinking about how far I've come. And I don't just mean how many miles I've totaled on that pedometer thingy. I mean over the last few years of my life, I have come leaps and bounds from where I was. I don't think it's all been my doing, although I have worked really, really hard to get here. I feel like God totally orchestrated this whole thing to happen. He triggered something in me so I would put myself out there and tell everyone who would listen all about myself. People always ask me, "How did you come to do this?" They just can't understand how a real person could get herself to where I was before *or* where I am now. The truth is, I not only owe a big thank-you to God, but I owe one to Helen Keller and Oprah Winfrey, too. I mean it.

One day, I was in my bedroom in the apartment I was renting on Fifty-second Street in Savannah, and I was flipping through the channels when I saw that the movie *The Miracle Worker* was on. As I watched it for the first time, it took my breath away! Here was a woman, Helen Keller, who could not see, hear, or speak. People had written her off; they called her dumb and treated her as if she was worthless. Then along came one person, a teacher named Annie Sullivan, who saw something more in Helen. She saw a person inside that shell, and she had faith in that person. I cried as I watched that movie. I really did. And then this unbelievable faith just came over me. This movie made me realize that the impossible really *is* possible. It made me see that the only limits we have in this life are the ones we set upon ourselves, and that one person's faith is enough to change the whole world. I thought, if someone with all of Helen Keller's problems, with all those things holding her back, could overcome her obstacles, then why can't I? I don't know why I happened upon this movie when I did, but it lit a fire in me—a big old barn fire that's still smokin' now. I really think God was trying to get my attention, and He did.

Not more than two days later, I was sitting at home, and this *Oprah* show came on about several severely obese women and their struggles. They were afraid to leave their homes because of the way society judged them. I have heard people call them shut-ins, but I could never use that word. It just makes me want to cry. I watched in complete pain. That show really broke my heart, because no matter what size I am now or ever was, I could never allow people to stop me from living and enjoying my life. Well, that was it! I knew I had to do something. So I called up my friends Jeff and Georgia and I said, "You need to get me a video camera. We need to document all of what I'm going through." Right then and there I had decided that I was gonna let people follow me around, step-by-step, so we could learn a thing or two together. Sometimes it just takes people seeing something with their own eyes to believe it. And that means me, too.

You know, in all my time at high school I barely cracked open a book. And when I went to college at Armstrong for two years, I was the biggest social butterfly. I never studied as much as I should have. Everything I ever learned, I learned by watching other people. You could call me a student of human nature. Somehow I thought that if we could videotape everything I did as I tried to lose weight, the world would get to see exactly what obese people struggle with every day. They could see us as human beings, not freaks or gluttons. They could see that something truly has a hold on us. And I could get to see what I was doing right and what I was doing wrong. While I was busy watching everyone else all those years, I'm not sure how closely I ever looked at myself. This was the perfect solution for *everyone*!

Georgia and Jeff were very excited. They knew that when I feel strong about something, there is no stopping me! And I was sure about this. In fact, I was never surer of anything in my whole life. Something had clicked inside me. I got the message loud and clear—and really that is how I got to be living this message now. It all started with some powerful TV shows and I guess it continues with my own show.

Here She Goes Again . . .

I used the word *helicopter* around someone today who didn't know I prefer saying that whenever I mean the place that's hotter than spicy southern barbecue. Another word I don't particularly like—though it's not a cuss, so I don't have a good substitute for it—is *doubt.* I think that word bugs me because I know it's what a lot of people had when I told them I was going to try to lose the weight again. It means a lack of faith or belief. I understood that it would be hard for some of my friends and family to take this whole thing seriously or to believe in me when they've seen me attempt to shed the pounds a thousand times before. It was hard for me to believe in myself then, too, because I had failed so much already. But I pray this time is different. I feel like I have a mission. And to keep that mission, there is no room for doubt.

I remember when me and my friends started recording my journey, we filmed my whole body, from head to toe, to show how big I was. I borrowed a friend's camera and we taped me walking, sitting, eating, and traveling. We caught people's reactions. I even let them film my workouts. I had Georgia, Jeff, Denny, and some other friends follow me with that camera at all times of the day and night. Sometimes we filmed four to five times a week. It was hard getting used to the camera being there at first. I felt all "neckid"! But I knew there was a greater purpose. I was trying so hard not to be self-conscious. I really made myself act naturally. This wasn't a movie or a TV show; this was and still is a real person's life.

When I sat down for the first time to watch the footage we shot, I was in shock! I could not believe how fat I was! It was so hard for me to even look at the screen. I was thinking, "Ruby girl, you don't walk, you *wobble*!" The truth is, I never felt like I was that huge before. I just didn't see it when I looked in my mirror. I think maybe you become numb to it because it's all a part of you. At that moment I could have given up; that would have been easy. I had lots of practice in that department. But I'm really glad I didn't. The camera didn't lie to me, so I couldn't lie to me either. It was an important thing to learn.

The End . . . Almost

I had to weigh in yesterday. I swear I still get "nerdous" every time *("nerdous" is so nervous that I actually act nerdy for y'all who haven't caught onto my personal language yet!)*.

Well, I hadn't lost a pound, not even when I was so good this whole week. I was so disappointed that I couldn't write about it at all last night. I don't understand it. I really don't, but I'm trying hard not to focus on it or let it beat me. I have to remember that I have had worse trips to the scale before.

For the longest time, I had no idea how much I weighed. Not even a good guess. No normal scale could handle me. Then one day I was at Memorial Hospital for a checkup with my mother, Chris, and Georgia and I said, "I need to know." So we went down to the basement of the hospital and they put me on a scale they use to weigh big crates and boxes on. A freight scale! There were all these men working down there with the forklift, and I'm thinking, "I am going to get on *that* scale?" I took a deep breath. The pointer went around and around and then it landed on 716 pounds. I just shook my head in disbelief. How did I ever let myself get to this point?

Most of the time, back then, I wore huge jumpers. They were more like tents than clothes, so I didn't have any idea. I was shocked; my mother was there, and she looked terrified, too. She said, "Ruby, you gotta do something." Well, I have always been big, and I have always tried to lose weight, but this was different. I started becoming a little overweight as a child—maybe about thirty pounds overweight. I was probably eight years old when it started. By the time I was thirteen, I was at least a hundred and fifty pounds overweight—losing fifty pounds here, a hundred there, but always falling between a hundred and a hundred and fifty pounds over the norm for girls my age and height. The older you get, the harder it is, so I never got ahead of this thing. And truth be told, I wasn't miserable like those ladies on *Oprah*. I was totally a hacky camper—someone who is "happy wacky," you know. I just loved my life. I was very social; I went out with my family and friends; I enjoyed going to the movies and dancing. But I was kind of living with blinders on. I never knew how much more to life there was . . . until I started to lose weight. I had just accepted my limitations in the world without ever thinking more about it. Without ever thinking, "What else exists out there for me?" I didn't ever let myself imagine other possibilities.

My mom was pretty determined to get me help once she saw that number on the freight scale. She realized, even before I did, how my health was deteriorating. She begged me to go to a doctor, but I was scared. I knew I was dying. I felt my body shutting down. I was so tired all the time. My blood sugar was up to five hundred. I could have gone into a diabetic coma. The very first time I went to the doctor, he said, "You are in skyrockets. All your numbers are outrageous." So I went on all this medication, and forty days later there wasn't much improvement, even with all those pills I was swallowing. When I went back to see him again, the doctor said he was gonna put me on insulin shots, too. I was like, "No, no, I'll be fine. I'm not sticking myself with needles." So he looked me straight in the eye and he said, "Ruby, you are a walking time bomb. It could be today; it could be tomorrow. I can't do anything else to help you. You have to do something to help yourself."

Well, I walked out of that doctor's office shaking. That was some wake-up call! I remember thinking, "I'm supposed to die. This is it. I can't beat this. I have tried. I have lived my whole life trying to beat this, and I just can't do it. I'm supposed to die young . . ." But then a part of me started arguing with myself, saying, "Ruby, you know that's not true. You're not gonna die and you're not gonna let all the other people like you die either. You have to beat this. You are *not* giving up." It's amazing sometimes what finally gets through to you. Fear is a good kick in the butt. And I was scared to death . . . literally!

I think the reason I didn't succeed before was that I was always trying to lose the weight for somebody else. I was doing it because of this guy who wanted to marry me, or for my friends or family who were begging me to because they love me and care about me. But this time, for the first time ever, I'm doing it for me. I'm doing it for Ruby. I'm doing it to get better. To get healthier. To live. I'm doing it because I feel like there's so much more I want to do in my life. I have this passion now that comes from deep down in my soul. I really want to help me, and in doing so, I want to help other people like me. It really is bigger than me now. Way bigger.

New Beginnings

It was hot as helicopter and sticky out today in Savannah, the kind of day where I just don't love walking outside, even though I know I have to get in my exercise. On days like this I really miss L.A. I lived there for eight years, and I could have stayed out there for the weather alone. I went because it's home to Hollywood, and the fitness capital of the world. I guess I knew if I was going to do my whole documentary thing right, L.A. was the place to be.

Jeff moved there first. Then a year later Denny and I followed. Everyone watched us filming at the gym, at restaurants, and at functions, too. Soon people started to recognize me. They figured out what I was doing and cheered me on. People were all curious about me; some people in "the business" even talked to me about how great the idea of a show around my mission was. A lot of people gave me advice on how to shoot and what film to use. I documented my life for several years before the show came out and in that time I lost two hundred pounds! But then I got off track. I didn't mean to and I'm not exactly sure how it happened. It's just like, everything—the camera and all—got pushed to the back of the closet. I focused more and more on Denny and forgot about me. It was stupid to abandon myself like that; but I couldn't see that that was what I was doing. When Denny came into my life, it all became about him. He was the center of my world. After I realized what happened, it took time—a really long time—for me to pick up again where I left off. Then my friend Brittany Daniel told her friend Tim Puntillo, who is a reality-TV producer, about what I had been doing, and The Style Network talked to me. They really believed in me. In a way, it was just like when Annie Sullivan believed in Helen Keller. They helped me pick up where my mission left off. They promised to let me show the world my passion. Now, every time I get an e-mail that says, "Ruby, if you can do it, I can do it . . ." I promise, my heart just fills up. I feel so grateful for the way things turned out, for the chances I've been given. For the people who helped make it all happen. Folks I meet all the time tell me that I keep them going. Well, they keep me goin', too! It has been a very long road for me. And there is still so much further I have to go. But I know I'm not alone. And that really helps me. There are so many people on this journey with me, and even though we all haven't met face-to-face, I know we're holding hands in spirit and giving each other the strength to fight this thing once and for all! I'm confident that together we'll do it.

So that's the backstory. That's how I got to where I am now. And there is no place I'd rather be.

2   UPS AND DOWNS

Fighting the Beast

I had a horrible headache all day. I'm not kidding, I woke up with a severe pounding in my head, and it just won't quit. I've been taking pills to get rid of it, but it's still hurting. The food they tell me to eat is "natty" (worse than nasty!). I'm craving *my* foods today. I'm craving things like sweets and salt. I'm trying hard to distinguish between being hungry physically and being hungry mentally and emotionally because I think, I really believe, that I'm satisfied. My stomach's satisfied with the food. But my taste buds are not happy. My emotions are not happy. My mental is not happy because I'm not getting what I'm used to. That, I am convinced, is the headache! It's all this change.

I hate putting myself through this. I feel like I'm in rehab and I have to beat this addiction. It has been kicking my butt for so long, and I just can't let it keep winning. I call it the Beast. I don't know what it is, or why it has controlled me for so long. Ever since I was young, really. I don't know where it came from or what it's about, but I know that it wins just about all the time. It feels like I'm in a boxing ring, and the Beast I'm fighting is the biggest monster you've ever seen in your whole life. Every time I fight it and I feel like I've got it pinned against the ropes, it sneaks up on me from nowhere and it throws me down to the ground and kicks me. It takes me forever to get back up, to crawl and stumble back onto my feet, and fight it off again. It takes everything out of me—all my strength—and I feel like I just can't get away from it. I feel like this Beast takes me to a place where I'm weak. But I'm sick of it winning. I'm ready to finally knock it out and never go back into that ring ever again. So I'm gonna go night-night now and get some rest so I can deal with it once and for all tomorrow. That's all I can do: sleep, wake up, put on my boxing gloves, and wait for the bell to ring again.

"I Love That Song!"

A friend of mine said to me today, "Ruby, did you hear the words to that Miley Cyrus song? It reminded me so much of you." And she told me that she's gonna e-mail me the lyrics. Well, before I even got that e-mail, I am in a car and the song comes on the radio. I am crying just listening to it, even though I had no idea this was the song she was talking about! It's called "The Climb." It is so beautiful. I want to meet Miley so I can tell her how much I love it and how it speaks to me. It's all about faith. About holding your head up high and believing in yourself even when it seems like what you're dreaming is an impossible goal. It felt like I was supposed to be hearing this now. First someone tells me about it, then it's right on the radio when I turn it on. There's that part in the song about climbing a mountain. It's not about how fast you get there or what's waiting on the other side, "it's the climb" that matters. For me, that's what this mission is all about. Not how fast the numbers on the scale go down or what happens when I actually lose the weight. I can't even wrap my head around that because I have never known what it is to be anything but big. Right now, I have to focus on the climb. It's all about the journey. I really need to take in what I am learning about myself on the way. I gotta keep moving on the path. If I stand still I won't get there. I can't turn back now, not when I've come so far. What I really gotta do is keep on climbing! I wish everyone in this situation could just climb their mountain, too. That they would just start today. Right now. This very minute. That they would realize there is no tomorrow. Because everyone with an addiction knows deep down inside that tomorrow never comes for us. I really wish they would just start climbing with me.

A Shout-Out to BIG Fans Everywhere:
A Letter to Miley Cyrus

Hey, Miley!

Y'all are a Tennessee girl, so I like you already! But I wanted to write to tell you that I am probably your biggest fan these days. (Not just in size!) I love your song "The Climb." The first time I heard it, I just about bawled. And I love you for being such a positive role model for children. I get e-mails and letters from kids all the time. I swear, sometimes when school buses pass me on the street, the kids start screaming my name. It must mean that something I'm doing is getting through to them. But you know what this feels like way more than me! When I started my mission, I never knew just how many kids are going through what I am. Ever since I found out, I've been wanting to reach out to them in a big way!

Obesity in kids has reached epidemic levels. Some estimates say that 15 percent of our kids are severely overweight and another 15 percent are bordering on becoming that. And two-thirds of these overweight kids will become overweight adults! The fact that those numbers have doubled and tripled during the past twenty years really worries me. These obese young people are gonna be at risk down the road for heart disease, high cholesterol, high blood pressure, diabetes, stroke, and several types of cancers. Not to mention all the mental stress that goes with being overweight. When you're a kid, it's way harder to deal with the other things that come with this disease. So many of them are depressed, scared, and lonely. They think no one understands what they are going through; they think they don't fit in with the rest of the world. Well, I do know what they all are going through! I have felt what they have felt and still do! I wanna tell them it's okay. You can fight this Beast! I'm doing it.

I am hoping to put together an educational program to help kids learn the things I'm finding out about eating right and exercising. I'm also hoping to start an awareness program for all kids—even those who may not have this problem—so they will be kinder, and better informed, too.

But I'm really writing today because I'm convinced that your song "The Climb" will speak to the kids I'm worried about in the same way it spoke to me. I wonder if you could give a shout-out to them every now and then when you perform it? It would mean a lot. It would make them really listen to the lyrics the way I did. It will give them encouragement and hope just to be recognized and to know people care. My friends from Rascal Flatts were in your movie and they think you and your daddy are good people. I sense that, too. So I hope y'all will think about this request and that you'll continue to be such an inspiration to kids (and to me, as I'm just a big kid at heart!).

Love, Ruby

Love Letters

When I told my bestest friends I was writing a book, they all wanted to help me. So they sent my editor these incred-ible notes filled with their memories of our times together, how we met, and the sweetest words about how much we mean to each other. I think they were hoping that their thoughts would provide some background, but what they wrote really made me cry! I just had to share them with y'all so I sprinkled them throughout this book. People touch our lives and sometimes it's hard to remember that we touch theirs, too. We are never on this journey alone.

FROM THE HEARTS OF BRITTANY DANIEL AND
CYNTHIA DANIEL HAUSER

One of the things I love most about Ruby is that she makes you believe that you can do anything in life. If you have a dream, Ruby will help you realize it. She believes in you even more than you believe in yourself. And she will fight for you like a lion! That's why I was so happy that I could help her with her dream, to get her show produced. I may have started her on that road, but she has taken it so far beyond anything I imagined. I am constantly blown away by her courage, her strength, her determination, and her love. I truly find her such an inspiration. She walks the walk. She is a role model for everyone, whatever their issue or addiction might be. She is living proof that you can have the life you want to live; you can change. I see her now and I am just bursting with pride. No one deserves to be happy as much as Ruby, because she brings such happiness to everyone who crosses her path. I am honored to call her my friend.

—Brittany

Every moment I spend with Ruby is a funny moment. Ruby is self-deprecating . . . she's definitely not afraid to make fun of herself—or of anyone else. But her joking is always in good fun. I don't think I've ever laughed so much with anyone more than I do with her. As we have all observed, Ruby has her own unique language. She'll make up words to take the place of ones she can't pronounce. They always make me laugh. Or when she doesn't like something you're wearing, she'll point to your outfit with the bull symbol and say "I love that outfit," which means BS. It's all meant to make you laugh. And her friends all know there is one important rule we have to follow when we take pictures with her: always shoot down on Ruby, not up. She'll have you standing on a chair in the middle of a restaurant to get a good picture of her. Ruby always looks her best . . . she's a southern lady and knows how to use that to her advantage.

I'm from the South as well, but my accent becomes even more noticeable when I get around her. She brings the southern drawl out of everyone . . . even if you're not from the South. Ruby's intoxicating . . . you pick up her mannerisms when you're around her (high-fiving all the time, holding hands everywhere you go with her . . .). She is very affectionate. You always feel very loved by her. And she has always held her head high. She has never let her weight stop her from living her life to the fullest. Ruby is one of the most real people I know and she can always tell when you're not being your true authentic self. She will never let you be anything else but your beautiful self.

Even though we live cross country from each other, she's been there in a second for me when I needed her. I'm so happy my sister Brittany Daniel, Tim Puntillo, and Style could help make Ruby's dream possible. As hard as it is to share your wonderful friend with the world, everyone needs a Ruby in their life to inspire them, learn from, and give them hope that anyone can overcome their own battles. I believe that Ruby should be a counselor . . . she always gives great advice. She is a wonderful cheerleader and reminds us that we deserve good things in life.

You'll never meet anyone like Ruby. She was been put on this earth to change lives. I don't think losing the weight will be all that she does to inspire others. There are many special tasks ahead for her and I can't wait to see them all unfold.

—*Cynthia*

3　　CRAVINGS

Medium-Size Wish List

I posted a wish list on my blog a while ago. I have a lot of dreams, but because they're different from other people's, I didn't really let anyone know what they were before then. But once you make that list, it really is amazing how it grows and what it says about you. Most people dream about meeting Mr. Right or winning the lottery or becoming famous. When I dream, I am small. Isn't that funny? And my friends tell me that when they dream about me, they see me small, too. I dream mostly about doing the things that other people take for granted. I put things on my list like soaking in a long bubble bath that smells like magnolias, or rockin' in a rocking chair, or curling up in someone's lap. Or sometimes I dream about the fun things I see my friends enjoying so much.

Like when Jeff and Georgia used to talk about how they'd go camping or fishing, I would think to myself, "I'd like to try that!" Or when I would see someone pedaling by on a bike, I'd close my eyes and imagine the wind whipping through my hair as if I were riding, too. That's as close to the real feeling as I was gonna get. In my fantasies I could almost feel the breeze on my face, but being that free only happens in my head. These things—as small and simple as they sound—are just not possible for people like me.

But after I made my wish list and read it several times, I decided that my dreams are a lot like the light at the end of a tunnel. If I can make just one come true, then I know there's hope for all of them. That's the way I look at this list now . . . with hope. I add to it from time to time. And as some of these dreams come true, I cross them off and add new ones.

Extra-Large Wish List (Newly Expanded to Include More Fun!)

- I want to be totally INDEPENDENT!
- I want to go to the White House and talk to the president. I want to tell him my ideas about helping America save money in health care costs and about how we should start a program to help our nation break its addiction to obesity. What if all the money we spend on diet pills and diet soda could go to educating people and to finding a real cure. How amazing would that be?!

- I want to go through one day of my life believing I can beat the Beast!
- I want to remember my childhood! I really do!
- I want to take a bubble bath.
- I want to go snowboarding.
- I want to ride a bike.
- I want to go horseback riding on the beach.
- I would love to backpack and see life in different countries. Y'all know I want to eat fresh pasta in Rome, but I think I want to see the Eiffel Tower and shop for perfume and sexy undies in Paris, too. I want to visit Japan and learn their health secrets. (I heard the Japanese have the lowest obesity level in the world!) I want to go to New York and see a Broadway show because I have a friend who said it takes your breath away to stand in Times Square in all those lights. And I would also like to bring food to countries where children are starving not because they are on a diet, but because there just isn't a lot of food.
- I would love to get a job helping people or working with children.
- My dad was retired from the air force and one of the things I remember about visiting him on the base was watching the men and women train, climb the walls, run through this maze of tires, and jump rope. I wish I could do the same. I would call it an opportunity course instead of an obstacle course!
- I want to go on a carriage ride. I think they are so romantic!

- I want to ride a bike through Italy (maybe even one of those cute Vespas!).
- I want to go hiking through Australia and scuba diving in Fiji!
- I want to get a body massage and not be "humidified" that I am lying there "neckid." *(Y'all know that "humidified" is kinda like a cross between humiliated and horrified, right? Doesn't that say it all?)*
- I want someone to truly fall in love with me and never hear them say, "Ruby, you need to lose weight," or "Ruby, you need to change this or that about you."
- I want to know what it feels like for someone to tell me that I am beautiful and really *think* I am beautiful.
- I want to lay on a couch with someone and cuddle.
- I want to sit on someone's lap and be held.
- I want to be able to kneel down on my knees to pray (that prayer would be about how grateful I am that wishes really do come true!).
- I want to see a play, concert, basketball or football game and be able to stay because I can fit in a chair. I can't ever go to events I am invited to because all the seats are too small.
- I want to be able to sit in *any* restaurant, play, movie theater, and car without worrying about inconveniencing anyone.
- I want to go to the beach and sit in a beach chair by myself and not worry about it collapsing under my weight.
- I want to go to an amusement park and ride all the rides—especially the roller coaster.

- I want to shop all day without getting tired. (And I want to fill up my shopping bags with clothes that fit me!)
- I want to sit in one seat on a plane and I want to be able to use the restroom.
- I want to be able to buy an outfit, shoes, and jewelry I like, instead of settling for whatever is available.
- I want to wear cowboy boots and be able to pull them up over my calves.
- I want to wear jeans and a tank top or a flowy little sundress with spaghetti straps and have people stare—not because I look big, but because I look so *hot*!
- I want to be able to get a haircut without going into the back room to find a chair I am able to fit in.
- I want to be able to get a manicure and pedicure without worrying if they have a chair. *(See a pattern here? Even a big gal's gotta sit sometime!)*
- I want to watch the sunset while swingin' on a porch swing.
- I want everyone to stop judging other people so harshly because of looks, income, education, color, religion, or anything else that makes them different.
- I want to travel state to state and meet everyone going on this journey with me!
- I want to lose this weight so I can yell at the top of my lungs, "I did it, I really did it, oh my God, I did it!" And then I can look in everyone's eyes and say, "If I can do it, then you can do it!" And they will believe me because I am living proof that it can be done!

- I want to be under two hundred pounds for once in my life.
- I want to live. I want to be healthy. And I want to grow old the way people are meant to.

I have lived, I have, but I just feel like I'll never enjoy the fullness of this life until I beat this thing. I wanna go to places I've never been. I wanna do things I've never done. I wanna make and take every opportunity I can. I wanna be the free spirit that I always thought I was. The free spirit I am in my mind!

Being fat is a lot like wearing handcuffs. You're in shackles all the time. You're a prisoner and you don't ever realize it, because you are happy to some degree. You're living the most you can live in the situation that you're in. So even though I did this to myself, even though I didn't have a clue that I was doing it when I did it, I simply have to undo it. Now that I know, I simply have to undo it. Whatever it takes, I have to undo it.

Hunger Pains

I feel myself wanting to cheat *so bad* sometimes. Right now, all I want is a Milky Way and some of those spicy barbecue chips—the forbidden fruit! It's as if the world is just ganging up against me, waving temptation in my face no matter where I turn. Fighting that temptation is a 24/7 job. I go to church and they have Krispy Kreme donuts there. I pass a Bojangles', and their chicken biscuits just start callin' my name! . . . For most people, temptation is not a dangerous thing. But I know if I cheat just once, I will be right back where I started. Guaranteed. (Don't do it, Ruby!) It is so easy to put the weight back on. And if I go off this diet, I will die. That's just it; I can't go backward. Even if I get so sick of the diet, I must remember: it's diet or die, plain and simple. I know I need to focus on the goal, not on what's on my plate. But that is easier said than done!

Pizza Envy

Georgia really feels bad that I can't eat certain foods—I know she does because I see it in her eyes. When we all went out to Vinnie's, she and Jeff and Jim all ordered pizza with double cheese. I swear I wanted to kill them! I know it's not their fault; they can't eat for me. Still, I am not happy about that cheese in my face! I understand that they don't have the addiction—I do. But I sometimes feel like I'm being punished. I feel like I'm getting a big old time-out. I have my little Hourglass package with me and they're all enjoying a delicious meal while I am poking around in that little plastic plate of lukewarm food. And what am I eating today? Quiche! I don't like quiche one bit; nuh-uh! I don't even consider it a real food!

The most tempting type of food for me is sweets . . . birthday cake is one of my favorites! I have this picture of me when I was two years old. In it, I was looking at this beautiful homemade birthday cake. My mom—the light of my life—must have made it for me. It looked like the most beautiful birthday cake a little girl could want. It had creamy pink strawberry frosting and little lilac and blue flowers. It looked like I was admiring it just before I was gonna run my finger over the edges to catch all the extra icing. I just had that look on my face, you know? The first dollop of frosting always tastes the best. I bet I got the biggest piece of all that day because I was the birthday girl. That must have been when my love of cake started, but I'm just guessing because I don't really know. Now, when I celebrate birthdays and everybody is done blowing out the candles and having their slice, I have to go and pour dish detergent on the rest of the cake so I don't eat it. I am *baaaad* around birthday cake. It's gotta be that icing. Or maybe it's just that I love a party?

Food is as real an addiction for me—as much as drugs are for a drug addict or alcohol is for an alcoholic. I'm serious. Dr. Bradley says that the messages in my brain are programmed to say, "I'm hungry . . . " all the time. It's like you know you're not hungry, but you're brain is still saying, "Feed me!" Practically anything and everything can set me off—a smell, a TV commercial, an ad in the Sunday coupon section. When the craving comes over me, it is as powerful as a tidal wave. But eventually it will stop. Especially if I eat every three hours and drink lots of water. I have to try to remember that when the urges overtake me. But when those urges are there, it's hard not to get swept away by them. It takes every ounce of strength I have sometimes to just let that food be. Like cake. (Okay, I'm obsessed with cake at the moment. The very mention of it just now got me going. See how hard it is?) But with so many people rooting for me, I can't mess up. There are a lot of people—really good people—who have invested their time and efforts into helping me on this journey. I simply am not going to let them down. How could I? How could I let myself down?

My Ten Most Wanted Foods

I put together a warning list for myself today. Everyone has something that makes them go weak in the knees. Most people can enjoy these foods and not have a problem. But people with an addiction like me can never stop at one serving. These are so yummy I've had to outlaw them for now!!

- Just one whiff of hot, buttered movie popcorn is trouble!
- Driving past a Wendy's is tempting, too. I can just taste that double cheeseburger (hold the onions!). Arby's, Bojangles', and McDonald's are tough, too . . . In fact, chicken nuggets are the most irresistible! Is there anything happier than a chicken nugget?
- Spaghetti is probably my most favorite kind of food. I love it! I could eat it for breakfast. I swear, sometimes I dream about a big bowl of spaghetti.
- The smell of food cooking on the stove—especially good old-fashioned southern food like fried chicken and grits. Or biscuits baking in the oven. Just heaven.
- Oatmeal cookies, fresh baked. The smell, the taste. Oh my

Lord . . . I have never been a fan of chocolate chip cookies. But oatmeal cookies are my weakness!

- A shopping trip to the mall. There's Savannah Sweets—their counters are filled with pralines, turtles, and fudge. Mmmm good. (I've heard that some shopping malls even spray the air to make it smell like fresh-baked goods so people will stop to buy them—how tempting is that?!)
- Oreos dipped in milk. Jeff and I used to eat so many, we'd get sick!
- My Thanksgiving dressing. I make it the best. I stuff the bird with it . . . and myself!
- Chocolate. Hershey's, Milky Way . . . heck, any kind of chocolate. I will not allow myself one itty bitty square, because I cannot stop. I am a chocoholic of the worst kind.

That's ten . . . but wait! I thought of more.

- Pumpkin pie with whipped cream.
- Georgia's mac and cheese from scratch. Sinful! I swear. When she makes this, the whole house just smells like a big ol' pot of bubbling cheese.
- Barbecue chips. Potato chips. Any kind of chips. I used to eat a bag every night . . . then chase it down with a Milky Way.

But now I am learning to love new foods. Some are so good I'm actually starting to crave them instead! To help me focus on my new favorites I made a list of them too. Try them. You might be surprised!

New and Improved Favorites

- Sea bass, salmon, mahimahi, seared tuna, and tilapia. Oh my God, these fish are so good! Why didn't anyone tell me before? Were y'all keeping it a secret?

- Couscous and artichokes. Not as natty as they look. Actually they're very tasty. I swear!

- Egg whites, steamed veggies, and grilled chicken. I'm proud to say that I've learned how to make all these things for myself.

- Oatmeal. It ain't no cookie, but it's still yummy and it's creamy, too.

- Black-bean burgers. Don't go telling me they're good for you. I just like them because they taste almost as good as a real burger.

- Edamame, eggplant, and asparagus. Before, I had no idea what to do with these things. I didn't know how to eat them or cook them at all. Now I love them.

- Salads. Yes, Ruby is eatin' her greens! They're not so bad, y'all! I like lots of different veggies in them—the crunchier the better. And I eat them now with very light vinaigrette instead of the old million-calorie ranch dressing I used to pour all over them.

- Fruits like apples and strawberries. Sweet!

- Cottage cheese. I think it's creamy! And it's got protein and fills me up.

I was first introduced to Ruby through a mutual friend. We connected immediately. She was very complimentary and loving and accepted me before she really even knew anything about me. I am a preacher's daughter and had a bit of resentment about it because I just wanted to be "normal." Ruby taught me that "normal" is relative and that you have to accept and love yourself for who you are.

Ruby has no idea how much influence she has on people. I have been deeply impacted by her charismatic personality and her acceptance of those who would be overlooked or "thrown away" by other people. She has a wonderful way of making everyone feel good about themselves. She has taught me to surround myself with people who I know have my best interest in mind, and to be kind to those who don't because it will come back to you.

My happiest memories are summers in Savannah at Georgia's dad's beach house, just hanging out with Rube and Georgia, being girls, dressing up, taking pictures, laughing and talking. I loved the visits she would make to California when we lived there. It was like a vacation whenever Ruby was around! She brought laughter, joy, and a sense of belonging to my life. She became part of my family and eventually everyone, including my mom and my aunts, couldn't wait for her to come. There is a proverb that says, "It takes wisdom to build a house, but understanding to establish it." You can be the smartest person in the world and have a lot of head knowledge about what you think a home should be, but unless you understand the people in that home, it will fall to the ground. I feel like Ruby has always understood me and that is why there is always a place for us in each other's home and heart. That is why our friendship has sustained for so long.

My saddest memory was when we were flying back from California. Ruby had been visiting and I decided to return to the East Coast with her for a few more days. She was at her biggest (around seven hundred pounds) and I sat near her for five to six hours in a two-seater in coach. It was very uncomfortable, to say the least. I felt angry, sad, and a little hopeless all at the same time. I was angry at her for not losing this weight that held her back from so many things; sad because I knew what a horrible feeling it must be to know that you are too big to sit with your friend in two seats on a plane. I also felt hopeless wondering if anything would ever change, and if it didn't, would I lose my friend forever? I have always been very honest with Ruby about my feelings and vice versa. If I didn't care, I guess I would have never felt these feelings. With that said, I am very happy for her that she is finally seeing hope in her dreams. She is truly living her calling. I pray for her constantly that she will not be tripped by temptations that come like a thief. I love her with all my heart.

—Danna

4 SOUTHERN HOSPITALITY AND CHARM

Savory Savannah

I have been taking these walking tours in different cities lately and I'm having the best time ever. So far I've been to Charleston, Atlanta, Daytona, Philadelphia, Washington, D.C., New York, Los Angeles, and St. Louis and have fallen in love with the people in every one of those towns. I can see what they like about where they live and why they are so happy to show off their landmarks, restaurants, theaters, and parks to me. Where we live says a lot about us. The South was such an amazing place for me to have been raised. All this makes me remember why I still like living here as much as I do. I love my Savannah; it's a beautiful city. I think my favorite part is the historic district, because it's like stepping back in time. The old churches with their bells ringing sound like heaven. Strolling around, looking up at the sunshine filtering through the giant trees draped with moss fills me with such joy. It is just so peaceful and beautiful. And the springtime in Savannah is truly breathtaking! I love it when Savannah College of Art and Design shows old movies in the park; I love watching the guys play rugby; I love watching couples stroll by, and I especially love watching the doggies play with their owners. Everyone tells me it's so important to get out and walk around. So I'm taking their advice and pretty much walking everywhere. But roaming the streets of Savannah is the best. Anytime I am feeling antsy or stressed, I get up and head out the door. In just minutes I feel better. I also love our funky little hangouts, like McDonough's where our gang gets together to sing karaoke. And City Market is great, too. It's where the bands play at night. I love listening to music at the Mansion! I love so many parts of Savannah: the Isle of Hope bluff *(Isn't that a great name?!)*, the drive to Tybee Island, riding through the squares of downtown and River Street . . .

Unfortunately, most of my favorite places also involve food (there's that pesky temptation again!). Vinnie Van GoGo's has the best pizza in town (they also have a great spinach salad!). And Sweet Potato's has the best southern food. It's true, the South is all about hospitality and, of course, that means feeding you VERY well (so I pity anyone who comes to my neck of the woods on a diet!). We have great, delicious foods that are only known to us southerners (or we just plain make them better than everyone else; just ask Paula Deen!). We serve things like grits, sweet tea, southern-fried chicken, collard greens, barbecue, and fresh fried shrimp right from our local waters.

With so many delicious specialties, people ask me all the time, "Do you think you would have gotten this big if you lived somewhere else?" Well, my answer to that is: I don't blame the South for making me overweight, though I do think the food I ate my whole life didn't help me any. I didn't come from a family of health freaks; I wasn't trained to eat a balanced dinner either. Barbecue chicken, mac and cheese, greens, corn, biscuits. That's pretty much the way everyone eats around here. Jeff and Georgia were also raised on the same southern food. And it is *gooood*. But not everyone in the South has weight issues—which should tell me something. It's not the food that's to blame for my weight issues. My habits are to blame. In the South, people are brought up to celebrate every life moment around the table. Everything that happens to us, whether good or bad, is talked about over food. The dinner table is the meeting place where people catch up. And while you're doing this, y'all have no idea of what is going in your mouth or how much of it you're swallowing. Well, at least I didn't have any idea!

One of the most important things I am learning these days is to be conscious of what I am eating. I'm really learning to take my time. When you're shoving food into your face, you can't possibly register what you just ate. Your stomach and your brain have no time to recognize that you're full! I am even a lot more mindful of the kinds of foods I eat these days. I went out with Georgia the other night and she had a steak while I

RUBY'S DIARY

had grilled fish and steamed veggies and I was okay with that.
I really was.

Georgia on My Mind

I was sitting here today, thinking about how long I have known Georgia. Southern women have a reputation for being sassy and opinionated. Scarlett O'Hara, Annie Oakley, Dolly Parton. That's me to a T. We speak our minds. And Georgia sure has heard an earful from me over the years. I have always called things as I see them; I have personally been known to say out loud what other people are thinking but are too afraid to say themselves! If there's an elephant in the room, I am the one who is gonna talk about it. And I see nothin' wrong with that. Maybe my friends don't like it when I say something they don't wanna hear, but they know I am gonna be straight with them. Georgia accepts that about me. She is my very best friend, sister, and soul mate. We met at church when we were teenagers. She had a huge crush on Jeff, and he and I were friends. The first time I met her, I remember thinking that she was a snobby little rich girl. She showed up to the movies with a fur coat on! Her father was a big shot in Savannah, a home builder. I was like, "Who *is* this snooty girl??" What I didn't know was just how quiet and shy she was. When she didn't talk very much, I read that as her being all stuck-up and full of herself. But I couldn't have been more wrong! The next time we saw each other, things were different. She talked more, and I began to see her sweetness come out. I loved her! Looking back, I can't believe I judged her on what she was on the outside, when it hurts so much to have people do that to me. I was going out of town the next weekend to visit Jeff at college, so I invited her to go with me. It was one of the smartest things I ever did. She was soooo happy! We went and had the best time. Since then, we have been inseparable. We have gone through a surprise pregnancy, a wedding, a divorce, raising kids, the death of animals, the deaths of parents, relationships, and lots more. We talk every day. She is a sister to me, and like sisters, of course, we sometimes get on each other's nerves. There is only one thing I would change about her and that is the way she procrastinates! She puts off very important and unpleasant things thinking that if she ignores the problem, it will just go away! But I know better than anyone that if you ignore a problem, it only gets BIGGER. She is still working on this, but until she really deals with it, it's going to continue to drive me crazy!

Sometimes I just want to beat her senseless! *(Don't worry, y'all, that's just our crazy love talk!)* It's like I wanna shake her and say, "Why can't you see what I see?!" But I love her even with this flaw, just like she loves me with all my flaws. I could not be doing any of this without her help. We fuss at each other sometimes, but that's because we know each other so well. Every day, I count her as one of my blessings, and I'm sure I always will.

RUBY'S DIARY

Another Ax to Grind

As I am sitting here writing about how I could just choke Georgia sometimes for not seeing how much she procrastinates, it occurred to me that there must have been times when she would have liked to take a pickax to me *(more crazy love talk!)* for not going on this journey sooner. She encouraged me before for sure, but she and Jeff recently told one of the show's producers that there were times when neither of them noticed how big I had gotten. And Georgia is a nurse, for God's sake! It's as if in the moments between wanting to knock sense into each other, we are all really one, willing to overlook each other's faults the way we just can't see our own when they're right under our nose. No wonder they both hold such a special place in my heart!

Just One Slice

Today I reached a milestone. Anyone who knows my love for pizza will recognize it as a big event, too. I actually asked myself: "Ruby, could you eat just one slice of pizza and then walk away from the table?" As I was asking this I was looking at that pizza in my mind; I was having a heart-to-heart with it. It was kind of like staring down the class bully. And here's what I said: "Yes, I believe I now could." That is an amazing feeling. I have to stop and really let it sink in. I feel like I am finally in control and being in control is something I have never known around food before. There was a time, not long ago, that I would have just felt defeated from the very first bite. I would have given in after just one taste. I would have said to myself, "Well, I'll just start my diet tomorrow; let me eat today!" I would have had a lot more than one slice. Now I know I can't just put things off for another day or lie to myself. I have too many people here supporting me—my friends, my trainers, my doctors. But even with them around, there is nobody slapping my hand when I reach for food. There is no one in my head saying, "Nuh-uh . . . you don't wanna do that!" Now it's me saying, "You don't wanna do that!" Now it's me stopping myself from taking a wrong turn. And I feel proud of myself for that. Really proud of myself.

I'm also really proud of Georgia and Jeff—they're both losing weight, too. Georgia lost twenty-two pounds and Jeff, he lost eighteen. Maybe they feel guilty about stuffing their faces with those greasy foods when they see how good I'm being. Or maybe they're just learning along with me. (Now there's a thought!) Georgia is cutting her portions and choosing healthier foods. I am also working her out with the new exercises that I am learning from my trainers (she whines a lot, but it's fun to torture her!). I am so proud of her and just so hacky for them both—for all of us! I really do think my mission is contagious and this is proof of it.

Am I Supposed to Eat This?

From the minute I started on my prepackaged meal plan, I was confused. I had never heard of or tasted some of this stuff in my life. I didn't know what to make of it. Some things sounded strange; others tasted just plain natty or had no flavor at all. But it was because I was changing my palate. I was so used to my southern-fried foods! I had never eaten these things, so my taste buds were screaming, "What is goin' on?" It took a while to get used to, but now those buds are a lot more sophisticated than they were. I am not craving all that grease, salt, or sugar I used to love! I looked back in my food journal and realized I have come so far. I know now that tilapia is a fish, not the name of a small town in Tennessee.

Here are some of the things I have been eating this week:

- Grilled shrimp Caesar salad with our low-fat Caesar dressing. I miss my ranch dressing. I have never touched shrimp that wasn't battered and fried before, but this really isn't so bad.
- Grilled lemon chicken on crisp greens in a light lemon oregano dressing. Chicken that's not fried? Lemon for seasoning? And not just in your sweet tea? I didn't know there were so many colors of lettuce out there. Why didn't anyone tell me before?
- Pesto shrimp served with fresh green beans. It's green. All of it is green. I guess I've got to bite my tongue and try it.

- Texas-style turkey meat loaf with espagnole sauce served with brown rice and mixed beans. Texas style? Well, I was excited for something southern. But I can't even pronounce the name of the sauce. Help!
- Grilled chicken breast; marinated in Moroccan spices and served with fresh cilantro and Israeli couscous. Couscous? The name alone makes me laugh. And I am beginning to see a trend here: grilled, grilled, and more grilled. Which is way different from my previous fried, fried, and deep-fried!
- Grilled steak and mixed-bean tomato chili served with whole-grain rice pilaf. A healthy chili? With no cheese or sour cream? For real, y'all?
- Coq au vin: breast of chicken in a light Burgundy-wine-and-mushroom sauce served with red peppers, broccoli, and baby carrots. I am told this is French food. No wonder those French girls are so skinny!
- Roasted chicken breast with southwest tequila-lime sauce served with wild rice blend and vegetable pilaf. Tequila? Now we're talkin'!

So many people ask me about this meal plan, I gotta remember to ask Dr. Bradley to write me something about it so I can share all the details 'cause I'm just learning about it. Some people even tell me that they can't afford to go on a meal plan like this 'cause it's just too expensive! Well, that's just not true. It should never cost more to eat less! Maybe he can come up with a Wallet-Friendly Seven-Day Diet Plan that people can do, too . . .

RUBY'S DIARY

A Note from Ruby's Physician

To All of Ruby's Supporters and Admirers:

Last year, through a stroke of good luck, we were thrown into the national spotlight. I never expected it, but when my associate introduced me to a five-hundred-pound, five-foot nine-inch patient named Ruby who had heard of our weight-loss plan and was convinced that if we were to feed her right she could lose weight, life changed greatly for her and things got even busier around here! She admitted she did not know what she was supposed to be eating, how to grocery-shop, or how to cook. While she knew about calories and the food pyramid in general, she had never really been taught about the latter in school and needed to be reaquainted with which foods had high and low values. She was on disability and had no money, but she was talking with a reality-TV production company about the possibility of shooting her struggle to lose weight. This was an unusual situation, but as you know by now, Ruby is a remarkably compelling individual; she draws you in like steel to a magnet! So we agreed to work with her. As many of you have seen on the first show, we explained to Ruby that she was going to die if she did not lose weight. It was the truth, not just TV drama. That's when Ruby began the Ourlife (formerly Hourglass) portion-controlled, prepared, and home-delivered meal program. For a variety of reasons specific to Ruby's situation, she was placed on our 1,200 calorie plan and was gently introduced to exercise. I ordinarily would have started a person her size with her health issues on 1,700 calories, but she felt strongly that she wanted to start at the lower calorie level. As you well know, it is hard to argue with Ruby when she sets her mind to something, so I agreed to at least try it her way, monitoring her response very carefully along the way. Two months passed and we were all pleased that Ruby was doing so well.

Ruby had had diabetes for a year and a half. In fact, when we started the diet she had an A_1c of 9.8, which means that her diabetes was out of control. She was supposed to be taking two medicines for this condition: one of these prescriptive medications was to be taken twice a day and the other once a day. We were clear with her that she had to be vigilant about taking these medications to improve her condition. Four months of dieting later, she had lost 60 pounds and her A_1c was down to 6.7. She had made remarkable improvements in the management and care of her diabetes. We were able to stop one of her medications at that time and her weight loss continued. Five months later, her A_1c was down to 5.7, which was now in the nondiabetic range! As of the writing of this book, we are a year from the start of her diet. She is down to 333 pounds! With all of her exercising, we've raised her calories to 1,500. Ruby's message is clear: It's NOT okay to be overweight. As you have heard her say so many times before: "We all have to conquer the Beast within." So, as America watches Ruby eat her nutritionally balanced meals and exercise, she is literally inspiring hundreds of thousands of others to do so as well. As for our long-term goal: Ruby wants to get down to 150 pounds and she will not hear from me that this may not be realistic. She fully understands that she will need cosmetic surgery in the future to remove excess skin. As for her cholesterol, she wants to just see what happens with her diet for now. So we continue to follow it off of the statin. We are so proud of Ruby and the work we are doing together! Because she and I often get letters from people watching the show saying that weight-loss programs can be expensive, Ruby asked me to create a cost-conscious seven-day meal plan for people; this can be found below, along with some valuable tips I shared with her when she first started our program.

Please remember that before starting any weight-loss or exercise program, you should consult your own physician. Everybody is different, and as I have noted above, Ruby came to us with her own set of unique conditions that needed to be monitored closely. I hope that what is included here is helpful to you.

Wishing you good health,
Dr. Paul Bradley

Tips from Ruby's Diet Doctor

1. **Set reasonable goals.** I told Ruby in the beginning, lose ten pounds, then we will lose another ten. If you aim too high, you set yourself up for disappointment. And that can lead to abandoning your diet.

2. **Calories count.** And *you* should count *them*. A calorie is

still a calorie, no matter what anyone tells you. Calories are a measure of the amount of energy in a given quantity of food. With Ruby, we needed to reduce the calories to less than she was burning in a day. We actually measured Ruby's metabolism in the beginning because she was convinced that it was abnormally slow. It turned out that her baseline metabolism was 3,300 calories per day!

Although exercise is an essential part of dieting, Ruby was too immobile in the beginning to do much, so her initial weight loss was a result of reducing her calories. As she became more mobile we had more leeway in the balance between calories and exercise in order to achieve significant results.

3. **Be prepared**. Make your meals ahead of time. Waiting until you get hungry is too late. Hunger will make you eat too much. One nice thing about having your meals ready ahead of time is the ability to eat them as soon as the hunger measure hits. We find that satisfies the hunger before it explodes.

From Dietician Kate Melei:
The Cost-Conscious Seven-Day Meal Plan

If Ruby were not on the Ourlife meal plan because of the related costs, this is the type of diet we might have recommended for her.

Day 1

BREAKFAST: ½ cup oatmeal with ¼ cup walnuts or 1 tbsp peanut butter.

LUNCH: Subway five-dollar footlong of turkey, roast beef, ham, tuna, or veggie. Have each sandwich with as many vegetables as possible on wheat-based bread. Eat half for lunch and half for dinner or save the second half for lunch the next day.

DINNER: chef salad with light dressings.

Day 2

BREAKFAST: 3 egg whites, ½ cup spinach (canned, frozen, or fresh) and 2 tbsp feta-cheese sandwich on whole-wheat bread or minibagel.

LUNCH: small grilled fast-food chicken wraps (McDonald's, Chick-fil-A, or Sonic). Or make it yourself with low-carb wraps, light condiments, and lean lunch meats.

DINNER: 1 cup spaghetti or penne pasta with ½ cup sautéed black beans; minced garlic and olive oil simmered in the black beans.

Day 3

BREAKFAST: 1 cup generic Cheerios or wheat puffs with added ¼ cup nuts, or 1 tbsp flaxseed and 1 cup low-fat milk.

LUNCH: tuna, egg salad, or peanut butter and jam on whole-wheat bread (brand or generic is good). Vegetables of choice on it or with it (carrots, celery, lettuce, tomato, cucumbers, spinach). A low-fat cheese (provolone, mozzarella, or low-fat American); 1 piece of fresh fruit or canned in light syrup or juice.

DINNER: egg quiche with vegetables and Canadian bacon (no more than a three-inch-width slice at the crust end).

Day 4

BREAKFAST: 2 pieces whole-wheat French toast with 2 tbsp jam, ½ cup applesauce on it or diet syrup.

LUNCH: light vegetable, chicken, or pureed squash soup with 15 pita chips or 15 wheat crackers on the side.

DINNER: 6 ounces grilled chicken, turkey, or fish with 1 cup frozen vegetables, sautéed or steamed. Add 1–2 tbsp Parmesan cheese or low-fat shredded cheese as a flavoring; ½ cup cooked brown rice.

Day 5

BREAKFAST: 2 pieces peanut-butter wheat toast with 1 whole fruit of choice (not juice).

LUNCH: low-fat cheese-and-vegetables quesadilla using wheat tortillas with salsa for dipping; ½ cup fruit of your choice.

DINNER: lean hamburger or turkey burger with melted Swiss cheese or mozzarella on a wheat bun and lots of vegetables; ½ baked sweet potato, cut into wedges.

Day 6

BREAKFAST: 1 light generic English muffin with 2 tbsp low-fat cream cheese and a fruit.

LUNCH: chef salad with light dressing or spinach salad with low-fat feta cheese, tomatoes, and ½ cup nuts of choice with light dressing.

DINNER: 1 cup turkey chili with low-fat cheese and 1 cup green beans (fresh, frozen, or rinsed canned).

Day 7

BREAKFAST: 1 poached egg with 1 light generic English muffin and a slice of Canadian bacon.

LUNCH: tuna, egg salad, or peanut butter and jam on whole wheat bread. Vegetables of choice on it or with it (carrots, celery, lettuce, tomato, cucumbers, spinach); apples, oranges, or canned light fruits.

DINNER: any frozen, canned (drained and rinsed), or fresh vegetables in a stir-fry with any lean meat (chicken, turkey) or any lentil in place of the meat.

Snacks (2 per day; one midmorning; one midday)
- Any light yogurt, generic or name brand
- Low-fat cheese with wheat crackers
- Sugar-free Jell-O or Jell-O pudding made at home (not the individual cups sold in supermarkets)
- Light or in-juice canned fruits
- Fresh fruits, buy seasonally for better prices and buy on-sale items
- Trail mixes—make your own by using a cereal on sale, nuts, and a dried fruit
- Sugar-free drinks—most of these can be bought in bulk to cut costs

5 MISSING MORE THAN FOOD

Why Can't I Remember?

The weirdest thing is, if someone were to come to me and show me a picture of my family, including me as a child, I seriously would not know who those people were. I do know now, of course, because I have been shown these pictures. But I would never have recognized myself. I would never have known about my childhood at all, except for what people have told me. I mostly have "feelings" but no real memories of anything before I was ten years old. It's odd that the last photo of me at a normal weight was when I was around that age. I don't know why I can't remember. The doctor said he thinks something horrible might have happened to wipe away those memories. He also said I do remember my memories on some level because I was there, but that those memories are hidden. For some reason I have blocked them out. I won't let myself recall them. A part of me is afraid of what will happen if I ever recover some of those memories. I do have many great memories of me as a teenager, though. I was very happy with my family. We had a very loving relationship. So I can't imagine why every memory before then is gone. But I do know this—I want my memories back. I know that I can handle whatever it was that happened. Of course I'm afraid, but fear will never stop me again! Now I find myself asking other people what they know about that time. Some remember my teachers. My sister can even walk around the same neighborhood my therapist took me to and recall names of people in this house and that house. But me, I am totally blank. I always feel like people are playing the biggest trick on me. Did I really grow up where they say I did? Are they just teasing me? How could I *not* remember?

I do know that I loved and admired my mom. She was, and still is, the light of my life. I wanted to be with her all the time. Beyond that, I have two memories and that is all. I remember my dad coming home. He was in three wars, serving in the air force. I remember him waking us up in the middle of the night and giving us these beautiful Japanese robes. I was so happy to see him!

My other memory is not a good one. I used to have this constant dream, a nightmare. I'm with my brother John, who I love, and these people are coming toward us with torches. They burn our whole house down, and all that is left is our bathroom. And my mom locked herself in. She wouldn't let us in. And these people with torches keep coming closer and closer. I can feel my heart pounding; I can't breathe. I am so desperate to escape, and I am so terrified!

I know that this diary is supposed to help me find answers, but there are times when it only seems to present more questions. And the truth is, I don't know the answers to any of them. I can't make them up either. I have to listen for the answers that ring true to my ear. I'll know the right ones when they present themselves. This is not a movie. It's real life. It's *my* life. And I just have to trust that when I am ready to know what happened, it will come to me. Just like when I was ready to lose weight and I was guided to take the steps that brought me to this point now.

You-Know-Who Keeps Callin' Me!

My past haunts me . . . in more ways than one. Denny is callin' and callin'! I can barely say his name around my friends these days without getting an earful of "Ruby, don't you dare go there again!" I tell you, I have to practically hide in the closet or the bathroom when I'm talking to him on the phone, 'less Jeff or Georgia get all over me about it. They just do not like him and there is no way around it. Georgia gets all red in the face and I can practically see the steam comin' out of her ears. I can't say I blame them for feeling like this. She is a true friend and Denny hurt me. He hurt me bad. But

I have gotten over that. I have gotten over him. I only wish that they could get past it, too. They are like my guard dogs! Every time he shows up, Georgia makes some little remark or Jeff rolls his eyes. It is so obvious that he is not welcome. I feel bad that they do this. They don't even believe that I'm over him—or trust me. What is up with that? I mean, they can say what they want, but I know that I am okay with my relationship with Denny now. I know where we stand. I will never forget what he did to me, and I will never go back with him. Even if Jeff and Georgia are convinced that I run whenever he calls. (I don't think I do, by the way. I'm just a sucker for the sound of that Harley comin' up the street. It's the bike I'm in love with, not Denny!) If they could, my friends would build a fence around me with a big ol' sign that says DENNY KEEP OUT! I feel sorry for him. I do. He tries so hard to get back in their good graces. But it's not ever happening. They don't trust him. I suppose that's okay, but I really wish they'd trust me a little more.

Where'd All the Romance Go?

Jeff and Georgia may be mad at Denny, but people on the street are pretty much of two minds on the subject. Someone came up to me today and told me I should give him a second chance. Other people have told me to cut the cord completely. Even on my message boards there are two camps: Team Denny and Team Kick Denny to the Curb. It's hard to believe it, but Denny and I were together for almost nine years. He was the closest thing I've ever had to a boyfriend. I know it wasn't a "normal" relationship—it was bizarre in many ways. It was missing the passion. I mean, we were incredible together, we had romance. But even after all that time, I really don't know what it's like to have a boyfriend. As I watched other couples, I guess I knew deep down that something was missing. I did all that I could. I made the romance, I worked at making things beautiful, I tried everything I could to help the relationship out. And he tried, too, honest to God. He loved me as much as he could. But men are attracted to the physical. He couldn't get past that. So he left, and when he did, it was horrifying. It was like somebody kicked me over and over and over again in the stomach, the chest, the heart. I mean *literally* kicked me with hard boots on. In fact, really kicking me would have probably felt a lot better than the actual pain that I went through. It just came out of nowhere. I had no idea. I had no idea that it was the end. Denny led me on. He made me think that he was leaving because I wouldn't lose the weight while he was still with me. But how could he think that leaving me was the answer? How could he think that he was doing this for my own good? He even told me that if I lost the weight, we'd get back together. Then he left: it was November 2001. He left me here in Savannah, and he moved to Myrtle Beach. We were both crying, but I think I still kept the hope in my heart that he'd come back.

He called me every day we were apart, every single day, telling me, "I made a huge mistake, I want us to get back together." And a piece of me believed him. He came and visited me on St. Patrick's Day. I think it was in 2002. I knew that he was coming, so I did everything I could to get my weight down. When he walked in, he told me how beautiful I looked, and he acted like we were getting back together—as if nothing had ever happened. Then I found out that he had a girlfriend that he'd been dating two weeks after he moved back to town! Well, that was it for me. That was the final straw, and the most devastating moment of my life. I was alone, really alone. It was not like I could go to someone else. It wasn't like a lot of people were breaking down my door! A lot of my friends, when they break up with someone or they're in a fight, they turn to someone else or they date until they can find a replacement. I had no replacement, not even a chance of finding one. Denny was my one and only.

So I was left to deal with the pain. That's all that remained of our relationship after all those years. Pain. It was me; my dogs, Foxy and Lucy; Benjamin, Zachary, and Jim, dealin' with the pain. Jeff was away; Georgia was involved with somebody else. And honestly, I just didn't want them to know how bad it was for me. I think Jeff feels responsible because he introduced us. Thank God for Brittany and Cynthia. They were so supportive. And for my babies, Foxy and Lucy, Jim, Ben, Zach, and Karen. But my Marcia, my best friend from California, was there at two or three o'clock in the morning, spending four hours on the phone with me, talking to me, helping me to deal and to move on. Thank God for my MarMar! She's an amazing friend, a truly amazing woman! Thank God for TV, too—for *Will & Grace*, *Friends*, *Frasier*, and *Sex and the City*. Because of those shows, I laughed and laughed and I was able to forget for a while. But that time of my life was just horrible. I stayed in my house, I didn't want anything to do with another human being. It was so crazy, the only people I wanted around me were my babies.

I wish I could say I bounced back in a few weeks or a few months, but it went on *forever*. For three years Denny kept calling me, making me promises. But he was also with this other girl for five years. And then, one day, I woke up in the morning, and I wasn't sad anymore. Just like that—the cloud had lifted. I got over it. I got used to him calling and saying, "Ruby, you're the only one that's ever loved me like this! You are so priceless, you're a jewel, la la la . . ." Those words don't even affect me now, I swear. It's not that I don't believe him, because I do. I do believe he loves me. And I love him. I am just not *in love* with him anymore, and I will never be again. The first time he came back to visit me I hadn't seen him in seven years. I was so nervous and excited! First, I heard him driving up on the Harley. My heart was beating so fast. Then I saw him outside of my house. There was some kind of sensitivity when I looked at him standing there, but the other feelings were gone. They were all gone. It was like I was looking at an old friend of mine, but the love I had for him once was no longer there. I do like being with him. I really do. We always laugh; we always have a good time. I love walking on the beach with him. I love going out to a restaurant with him. We have history—that's not gonna change. We have a deep connection, and I just can't be mean to someone who was in my life for as many years as he was. I love Denny. We have a special bond that no one can break. We are what you call friends in love, best friends for life. We know each other inside and out and take our good along with our very worst.

I truly believe in soul mates. And I believe that mine is out there. I just haven't been able to meet him yet. Sometimes I wonder if, because I've been fat for so long, my soul mate could have been taken already. But truthfully, I don't wanna be with anyone else right now. I don't wanna settle. When I find Mr. Right, I'll know him, like I know the color of my own eyes. I just don't want to be with anyone in this world because I'm lonely or desperate or whatever. That's just wrong. I'm happy with Ruby. I'm happy with Foxy and Lucy. I'm happy with my friends, I'm happy with my family. Would I love to have love, like in the movies? Yes. Would I love to find that perfect guy, that perfect soul mate who loves me for who I am on the inside, not the outside? Yes, I would love it. But I'm not gonna sit here waiting. And I'm not gonna wish for something. If it's meant to be, then it's meant to be and it'll happen. But I'm not looking for that right now, at all. All I'm looking for is to fix Ruby. Ruby's gotta be fixed first. I've gotta do it for myself and no one else. If I lose the weight, it's not because Denny or anyone else gave me an ultimatum. It's because I am ready and I want to do this for me.

This last time, when Denny said what he said to me—"we could still have the dream, we could still be together"—I felt so sad because I could see it in his eyes. He believed it. He meant it. He really did. Now, the last thing I ever, ever want to do is hurt anyone. But I just don't want him anymore. It's not like I want to hurt him like he hurt me. I don't want revenge. I just want to put myself first for once in my life. And if I lose the weight and Denny realizes he has lost the best woman that he will ever find, then I am sad and sorry. But that train has left the station.

When people ask me why I don't date, I say, "It's not like I have people asking. Remember, I am the fat girl. Guys just don't go there except as friends." Even if I was asked out, I just gotta tell the truth: it's hard for me to even think about it. I don't wanna go through the hurt again. Right now, for the first time in my life, I am falling in love with me! And that's not such a bad thing.

There's a Comfort in Being Fat

I wasn't feeling well today, so after I watched the movie *Sleepless in Seattle* for a while, I decided to go to bed early and snuggle under the covers. I know people say all the time that weight is like a security blanket. I've said it myself, but as I lie here covered in my quilt, I really know what that means. My body, the way it is, is all I've ever known. I can understand when people say they're scared to lose weight. There is peace and comfort in something that is so familiar to you—until somebody shows you something else that can provide that same feeling. Sometimes I wonder, "What will I look like small?" When I look at a normal-size person's arm, I'm always thinking, "There is no way my arm will ever be that size." I just cannot see myself like that. So it does scare me to imagine that one day, that could be me. I want it to be me. I want to be normal so I can do so many more things.

I have a friend who lost a lot of weight. She's nearly half her size now, and she tells me that she couldn't recognize herself when she looked in the mirror. For a split second, she thought, "Wait . . . who is that?" The whole time now, she's feeling like a big ol' liar. She's thinking, "I'm not really this skinny girl. There's a fat one here inside." I feel sometimes like I am grieving; I am losing my best friend—the *big* me! It is so mental. People think that weight is all about eating, and I swear it is not. So much of it is about how we see ourselves in our own minds. There is a reason I am this big. I haven't figured it out yet, but I know it is a very real reason and it has nothing to do with what I eat. When I was on Oprah's show, she turned to me during the commercial break and said, "Ruby, what are you feeding?" She understands. She knows that when you're overweight, there is something you're missing or wanting in your life. I try so hard sometimes to figure it out, it makes my head hurt! I think I'll just turn out the light and go to sleep 'cause I can't think about it all anymore right now.

FROM THE HEART OF MARCIA THOMPSON

I met Jeff through a mutual friend out in L.A., and he would often speak of his longtime friend and roommate Ruby. One

RUBY'S DIARY

Sunday we were all in attendance at church. She came up to me and introduced herself. I reached my hand out to shake hers, and she grabbed me into this big bear hug. I was taken aback just a bit because it was like she knew me. But we all went out to lunch and she and I have been friends ever since. I also remember I was driving Ruby someplace, and we were talking. I hadn't known her that long, and she reached over to hold my hand. I tried to withdraw my hand discreetly, but Ruby just held on. We kept talking, and she could see it on my face that I was thinking this to be strange. Of course, now that I know her so well, it's just who she is. I've said to her often, "Jeff couldn't have prepared me for you!"

Ruby is warm, funny, friendly, bossy, compassionate, caring, stubborn, determined, faithful and faith-filled, tolerant, a peacemaker, frustrating, intuitive, and encouraging. She will be your "biggest" cheerleader if you have a dream or goal. And if you don't have one, she will tell you what your goal or dream should be based on her intuition and understanding of the person she knows you to be. She makes it easy for you to be yourself.

I have been through a few sad times with Ruby: her dad dying was the most recent. He was a big part of her life. She loved, admired, and respected her dad. Then there was the breakup with Denny. I've never, including my own divorce, felt so much pain. I could feel the hurt through her voice. It was horrible. Then there was the time when she left L.A. I didn't get to see her every week, so we were both bawling!

But for every sad time, there have been a hundred funny ones! There is the bench story. I really must tell the bench story.

There was a movie theater we would go to all the time in L.A., and they would bring an armless chair for Ruby to sit on. Well, one day, we went and the chair was missing. Management couldn't find it, so Ruby and I waited inside the theater for Jeff to bring a replacement. When the doors opened, Jeff and one of the movie attendants were carrying in a long bench from the lobby area. Here the three of us are, sitting on that bench, watching a movie. I whispered in the dark, "Ruby, what has my life come to that I'm in a movie theater on a bench eating popcorn?" We laughed and laughed.

Another time, Denny had gone out with a friend. He told Ruby the place he was going to had just recently opened and he wasn't a hundred percent sure of the name or the address. Well, it got late and Ruby was worried, so she called me and together we set out to find this place. We drove through Hollywood on a Friday or Saturday night looking for it. The streets were packed, but Ruby was determined. Up and down the streets we went. I told her, "If Denny sees us, I'm going to be so embarrassed. We're spying!" I'd given up, but not Ruby. We were sitting in a far lane waiting on the light to change when Ruby spotted a newsstand. She yelled out of the window in that sweet southern voice to the vendor and asked him if he had a weekend paper. He yelled back yes and then proceeded to run it to her. Only Ruby could inspire somebody to run across traffic and risk life and limb. You'd do that for her.

Needless to say, Denny was okay and Ruby's escapade gave us both something to laugh about later.

—Marcia

6   A CHANGE IS GONNA COME

Back to Work

A few weeks ago I decided that it's time. I am ready to get a job and go back to work. I had been working nonstop ever since I was sixteen, and I really liked working. Then several years ago the doctor told me I couldn't work anymore, but now I feel like I can do it again. I'm ready. I can stand on my feet; I can move around. I can contribute! When I told Dr. Bradley, he got real quiet. "Are you sure, Ruby? That's a big step." I think he wanted to see if I would stick to my guns; if I was really ready or if I was just throwing the idea out there. He looked worried. And that didn't give me a whole lot of confidence. Maybe he knew what I was in for?

At first, everything seemed great. I started sending out my

résumé and I would always get a callback. Each time, I would talk to the person who was doing the hiring for almost an hour, and I always heard it in their voice—they could not wait to meet me. They wanted to hire me right then and there on the phone! But when I would show up, I could see the shock on their faces as I walked in the door. They'd look me up and down; one even shook her head and said, "Well, I'd be worried about the insurance risk . . ." I was mad at her, but at least she was honest. Most just lied to my face: "Sorry, we hired someone else already . . ." I investigated a few times. I sent a friend in later to ask about that job and I found out that it wasn't true. No one else had been hired yet. The position was still open. So why not hire me? I'm the same person you chatted with on the phone, the same qualified person on that résumé paper. Do you really think my size changes all that? That's plain ol' prejudice, and I see it everywhere. My weight does not define me. That's not all of who I am. I have great parents, great siblings and friends. And they love me. I have great life experience, too. And I am good with people.

When I was a teenager, I dealt with parents asking their children, "Why do you hang out with her? Aren't you embarrassed to be seen with her? Do not let her sit on our furniture, do not let her in our cars. She'll break them!" When you're obese, people treat you differently. They look down on you. I try to understand where they're coming from, I swear I do. I try not to judge them the way they judge me. I really do give people the benefit of the doubt. I try and imagine what it must be like to be them, looking at me. I know it has to be hard to

RUBY'S DIARY

see someone who is seven hundred pounds, or even four hundred pounds and understand. I can't sit anywhere I want; I do not move around fast. I am abnormal-looking in a society that doesn't have a lot of Rubys. I know when I walk into a room there has to be a little shock factor.

But I really wish people didn't make assumptions about me. They come to the conclusion that I am overindulging in foods. That I don't care about myself. That I'm slow or lazy or there's something wrong with me because I have let myself get into this situation. They can't grasp it. But once they get to know me, they are different; they see Ruby finally, and not her shell. I just want to tell them I know, I really know. I am just as confused as they are. I do not understand how I got here either. I wish they could walk my path with me, fit into my soul, and know where I've been. See how I've been trying to save myself for so long.

No matter how many harsh words I hear—or how people misjudge me—I still do believe that there are more good people in this world than bad. And some of those bad people are just scared or insecure. They usually come around in the end. But there is something I wish I could say to them before that. I just wish I could tell everyone, "When you look at a Ruby, please, please, please show some compassion and remind yourself that we all have our own Beast we battle. I just wear mine on the outside."

Intolerance is a Beast, too, you know. And it's as visible as my size is. It can be very ugly. I would see it in the way people looked at my brother John sometimes. He is an angel; a beautiful person, an innocent pure heart, a man-boy who loves unconditionally. But he is mentally challenged and there were people who only saw what was different about him. Not the good. If my mom passed, I would take John in with me, and we would live together and grow old together! I am very protective of him.

As a teenager, I took John everywhere with me—and I mean everywhere. He's six-four and loud, and he would draw stares and unkind remarks from total strangers all the time. They didn't even know him and they would do that. I would get so mad, and I would defend him because he couldn't defend himself. Georgia and Jeff would be with me, and they'd say, "Ruby, let it go. Don't go there. Don't sink to their level. They are just ignorant. They're the stupid ones, not John." It would take a lot of strength sometimes for me to turn my back and walk away. But they were right. I see that now.

Seeing the mean side of some people, I became a big believer that your brain can be your worst enemy or your best friend. You can listen to somebody's opinion and make yourself believe it; or you can find a way to turn it off, to listen to the voice inside your head, the voice that knows the truth, not all these hurtful lies. And you have to remember that you never know who is gonna sabotage your dream; sometimes it's not even a stranger. It can be a parent, a sibling, a friend, a teacher who will try and tell you something to kill your passion. And you won't even realize it, because you will think that these people know you and have your best interest at heart. Well, if you go letting someone do that to you . . . you have to ask yourself, "Who is to blame?" The answer is simple. You! Everyone is here for a purpose and has a destiny. If you have a passion and it burns inside you, that's what you should be doing. Is the road ahead gonna be hard? Yeah. But the hard road is the road that will lead you to the right place. I know. I really know.

And those jobs all those people turned me down for? Well, they don't know what they're missing . . .

The Christmas Doctor

Dr. Bradley tells me I need to go see the gynecologist. I need to have a breast exam, a mammogram, and some other stuff. None of it sounds good. It's important, he says, for all women my age to do this. Well, I am just not a hacky camper at all about this. In my whole life I have gone to the "Christmas" doctor two times; it's uncomfortable, it's humidifying, so I avoid it. It's really embarrassing! I can't even call it by its right name. I call what's down there Christmas—because I think of it as a gift you give only to a certain person like your hubby. It's a nicer and sweeter thing to say. And Dr. Bradley wants me to go for an exam? When I can't even say the word? I don't know. I just don't know if I can do it . . .

Bribing Georgia

Tonight when I was out with my girlfriends I asked them how they feel about going to the gynecologist. I don't mean to be obsessing about it, but I guess I am. Have they done it? Should I go? They all say yes; it's not so bad. I trust them; they wouldn't lie to me. Still, I need some backup. I convinced Georgia and Leslie that they have to go with me. Georgia gets all "nursey" on me; she was just not gonna let me get off of this one. She's all, "Ruby, you *have* to go!" She can't understand why I am so shy and sensitive about the whole thing. She thinks I should be more easygoin' about it because I have these pretty, sexy bras which I like to wear all the time. I don't see what one thing has to do with the other—but Georgia seems to think they are related. I have sexy undies because if you're wearing something sexy, you just feel good about yourself. And there's not many sexy things I can find, so when I do, I indulge. I love it. I buy as many sexy bras as I can find. Well, I told Georgia I would go to the doctor if she let me buy her a bra that is sexy. It would make us both feel good about doing something that didn't seem like much fun but is so important for our health. And she said okay—but I don't think she really believes I am gonna keep her to it. I will! I am so nervous about this checkup. I'm not sure what scares me more—knowing I am going to be laying there, all exposed, or the fear of what they'll do to me while I can't see what's goin' on! Or maybe I'm afraid of what they'll find.

Testing Positive for Strength

Well, going to the Christmas doctor wasn't as bad as I thought it was going to be. Georgia and Leslie held my hand and it didn't take more than maybe five minutes before the whole thing was over. So I guess your mind builds things up to be a lot worse than they actually are. The doctor was real nice; she didn't make me feel embarrassed at all. Then she says she has a present for us—and I'm thinking, "Ooh, do we get a lollipop? A free sample of something?" Nuh-uh! She is going to give me, Leslie, and Georgia a mammogram, too. Then she sent us over for it. Lord, you should have seen Georgia's face. She was whiter than a ghost. She is terrified of mammograms. Leslie got out of it because she's still "breasticle" feeding *(I can't say that other word either . . .)*.

I went first and it didn't hurt at all, but I could see Georgia's face through the window. She was so scared. She's just standing there, waiting her turn, watching them do it to me. I'm goin', "Y'all, this does not hurt!" but she is sweatin'. I felt bad for her because I know how she feels. It's how I felt with the gynecologist. Now she's in my shoes! I thought she was gonna run out the door, I swear. I could see her looking around: Where's the exit? But she didn't run away; she did it. And I did it. I'm proud of us both. Truly, there was nothing to it. It was good news and I had such peace of mind. I will never be scared of it again. And neither will Georgia! Everyone has to face their fear sometime. There's power in it; there's peace in it. I think when you conquer one fear, it gives you strength to deal with something bigger down the road. I guess I'm getting stronger every day.

My first impression of Ruby was that she was more than a little crazy. When I was growing up, my family was loving but not very affectionate. Well, Ruby is a hugger. So she's hugging me, and I don't even know her. It was shortly after Jeff introduced us that I was in the mall one day. She was coming out of Pancho Taco, and she screamed from about fifty feet away: "Oh, Georgia! Come to Mama!" Here is this big girl, with her arms out, screaming my name in public! That's just Ruby. I got over the humiliation, and we became the best of friends.

She would embarrass the crud out of you if she thought you liked a guy. If there was a cute one driving by, she would hold your head out the window! She would get us in so much trouble—but she has a mind like a machine. She can think so fast that she'd get us out of trouble as quick as she could get us into it!

She's a magnet. I was so attracted to her zeal for life. She always looked nice, always so pretty, and she always smelled so good. You smell Curve perfume or Chanel and you think of Ruby. She wears the sexiest Victoria's Secret underwear, and she has such a fashion sense. When we were younger, we'd get all the style magazines, and she would cut out all these pictures of these girls she wanted to look like. I went on all the diets with her. Atkins, The Zone, the Ice Cream Diet. We had cabbage soup coming out of our ears and noses.

She has a sixth sense. She has an unbelievable perception of people; she can read you like a book and she will know who you are, if you're for real or if you have an agenda, within five minutes. She's 95 percent accurate on this.

She's probably the wisest person. She thinks and doesn't make rash decisions. I know, even though she's uneducated bookwise, she has the most smarts of all of us. She is a nurturer. Kids love her and are drawn to her. She has bright eyes and a bright face and they see her goodness radiating from within. You can't BS a kid. They see right through you.

Ruby changed my life when she came into it; I can't imagine my life without her. She wants to find me a soul mate. This is like her mission, God help me! But she's my soul mate. She knows me in and out. She knows I hate confrontation and I procrastinate and I pay my bills late. There are things about her that bug the crap out of me—like if you don't do something just the way she wants it done, she's yelling her head off (then apologizing five minutes later).

She says all the time that we're her support team, but she is ours! I couldn't have survived divorce, a breakup, dating a jerk of a man for seven years, going to nursing school, losing my dad, or being a single mom without her support and love. If I hadn't had Ruby all those times, I wouldn't be here today. After God made her, He broke the mold.

I have told her how thankful and happy I am to be here doing this with her. It's a thrill. I am not only grateful for the process of doing a TV show, but for finally knowing that I'm going to have a healthy, skinny girlfriend. I just don't know if I can hang out with her when that happens . . . you know, she's gone be freakin' gorgeous . . .

Ruby, you are a light to a dark world.

—Georgia

7   MY HEAVY HEART

I Miss My Daddy So Much

My daddy, James Edward Gettinger, is gone and my heart aches in ways I have never felt pain. I could cry right now—and you'd think that I would be all cried out at this point. But the tears keep coming. He passed away on January 13, 2009. He went into the hospital, just before Christmas, and he was there for about two weeks. When they let him out shortly after that, I thought, "He's doing good again, he'll be okay." I'm not sure I believed it, but I wanted to. I wanted it to be so because it had always been that way. My daddy was a survivor. I remember him lifting these big bar weights. He did this every single night, and it kept him in shape. I'd watch him lift them, up and down, up and down: the strongest man in the world.

He wasn't able to walk at all for the past ten years because diabetes attacked his nerves, and his legs didn't work anymore. My mother always stood by him a hundred percent, taking care of him, helping him, right up till the very end. And me and my siblings, we tried to help her, too. After being in the hospital those two weeks, he just wasn't the same. He was in and out of consciousness; I may have gotten five minutes of him, because he slept most of the time. He was so filled with toxins (the doctors said he was septic). His leg was getting worse and worse, and he had to go back into the hospital on his birthday, which is December 28, the day he turned eighty-one. I got him some gifts, but he only opened his eyes for a total of two minutes to see them. It makes me sad, 'cause he never got to enjoy his Christmas presents or his birthday presents.

When they took him back to the hospital, just about everything you could imagine was going wrong. They needed to give him kidney dialysis. Then the doctors said they had to amputate his leg and he wasn't even awake to know that they were doing it! He wasn't even able to make that decision for himself. But it was either that or he would die. I remember they were taking him to the operation, and my sister Jamie was on one side of him, kissing his forehead and saying, "I love you, Daddy," and I'm on the other side of him saying, "Daddy, you fight this, you beat this! You're coming back. Don't you worry . . ." He and I have always been the fighters in the family.

Well, then he opens his eyes and says the last thing he ever said to me. He goes, "Ruby, you gotta get off me, you are so heavy." I said, "Who tells their child they are heavy? That is uggy, Daddy. . . ." Then we both smiled, because we were jokin' each other. My dad had never once said anything about my weight, anything at all. Never said I was fat, never said I was too big, he was never embarrassed of me. This man loved me.

He came out of surgery, and I went through helicopter because the first thing they said to us was "He's not waking up." Well, he proved them wrong and woke up. So I went home to get a little rest, and the next thing I know, I've got Georgia and everybody calling me saying they just did CPR on him. They brought him back. After that, I was afraid to leave his bedside for even one minute! Every day, the doctors would make me leave: "Ruby, go home, go home. He's fine, we will call you . . ." I was so tired, but I wanted to be there for his last breath; I didn't want him to be alone. None of us did. And every time we did go home, someone would call: "Get over here, he's not gonna make it. Hurry up." Every time that phone would ring, I felt like I was having a heart attack.

So for three days and three nights, I didn't sleep. I didn't sleep at all. And my meal plan had gone out the window at this point. Not totally: I ate the breakfast, I did a couple of the fishes. The chicken . . . but I just didn't wanna eat. I wasn't cheating; I walked by a vending machine in that hospital every single day, every single night, every single morning. And I wasn't even tempted. I didn't want anything. I saw the candy and I saw the chips and I was like "It's not worth it." But I wasn't working out; I wasn't thinking 'bout myself. I didn't care about any old diet. I didn't care about anything except making sure Daddy lived. And I was wor-

RUBY'S DIARY

rying about my mom: Was she gonna be okay? My sister, my brother, my nephew, my niece, how were they gonna handle this?

Then finally, they called us in and said, "He's gonna leave today. It's not gonna be long." I'm going, "What do you mean? What happened?" But there was nothing more that could be done; he was totally on a ventilator and they said his heart would flatline. They actually thought he was gonna die three days before, but he was fighting so hard.

So we were just sitting there and they said, "He's gone." Just like that. I looked at him, and he seemed so peaceful, like he was still just sleeping. I laid on him. I was rubbing his head, his neck, his chest, kissing his face. I didn't want him to turn cold, so I put a towel on his head. I couldn't let go. I felt like if I did, he was gonna be so cold. And I couldn't bear that thought.

He had a beautiful military funeral. They talked about him fighting in three wars: World War II, Korea, and Vietnam. He was dressed in his air-force blues, and he had all his medals on; he was a senior master sergeant and he served over twenty years. It would have made him proud to be sent off this way. He was a good, good man. People—they mean well— they kept coming up to me and saying, "Ruby, he's in a better place now . . ." I know my daddy is with God and pain-free. I know he is in a better place. But I do not want to hear all that. Why? Because I want my sweet, gentle daddy back with me. I want to see his face and hold his hand. I want to hear him say, "Hi, baby!" No matter what he was up to, when I walked in the room, his face would light up and he was beyond happy to see me. We would talk on the phone three to four times a day. And every holiday when midnight struck, we would race each other to see who would say "Happy Birthday," "Merry Christmas," or Happy New Year" first. No one ever called me baby but my daddy. When he said that, it made me feel happy and at peace. I trusted him like no other. He never lied to me. I was so proud of him for serving his country. He always worked hard, and he made sure we had a roof over our heads and were always taken care of.

I never ever heard him complain about ever having to go to work for twenty years at the U.S. Postal Service. Even when he got home at night and he was exhausted, he never moaned or groaned or complained. He worked in his shed making furniture, and toys, too. When I got to be my biggest, my dad knew I couldn't fit in many chairs, so he made me this huge wooden one that when I sat in it, I felt so tiny. He was the most giving man I knew; he would give you the shirt off his back. I never heard him swear or curse. I never saw him drink or smoke. He practiced what he taught me.

He loved us all so unconditionally. He loved everyone that way, and he never said an unkind word toward anyone. My mom was his soul mate. If ever there were two people that were meant to be together by the hand of God, it was Daddy and Mom. They knew each other only a month and were married fifty years. I can truly say I have never seen a man love a woman the way my dad loved my mom. In his eyes, she could do no wrong. They were always laughing; he was always holding her hand, grabbing her to hug or kiss her. She was his queen and he was her king.

My daddy was a man who was strong, but he grew the prettiest, most delicate morning glories you ever saw. He had his own garden in the backyard and he would grow the biggest cucumbers and tomatoes. He was a man who loved sports so much he would watch one game on TV and have earphones in his ear listening to another. He was a man that could fix any vehicle and taught my nephew Jim the same. The best times for my daddy were working on the car and teaching Jim. His grandchildren were the joy of his life.

Everyone is hurting over losing him, but I am a mess. I don't wanna eat. I just want to sleep, sleep, sleep. I have been wearing his sweatshirt, his flannel shirts, lovin' them, lovin' him. The treadmill is right there beside my bed, and I can't even get up to use it. I have not an ounce of energy. I just don't care. The last thing I want to do is exercise. I haven't even been following the meal program for three weeks. I am worried— and so is everyone else—that this is it. I am never gonna get back on track. I can't get on the scale. I am so freaked out. Jeff is trying to be all funny: "You gotta dust cloth for that thing? Time to weigh in!" But I can't face the possibility that I gained one pound, much less more.

Finally (thanks to everyone bugging me) I stepped on the scale. And it says, "365.8 pounds." I gained 5 pounds. That is a wasted month. I was trying so hard to get under 350. Then all this happened, and all I can think is, "Here I go again. Here comes the weight back!" I am in a rut; I just want to see my dad. I just want to get in my bed with a big ol' bowl of spaghetti. My friends, they are trying everything, but I just can't shake it.

Denny to the Rescue

Last night Denny called me. He has this sixth sense about when I need him. Truly. He knew that my father had just gone, and he wanted to come to the funeral. He called every day, wanting to come be there for me, making sure I'm all right. I told him, "Denny, that's a bad idea. It's gonna be too much stress." It's already stressful enough what's going on, and my friends . . . well, they like him, but they don't like him. I feel bad telling him not to come, but I don't need to be hearing it from everyone if he's there. I can't handle it right now.

So he waited a week before calling me again. This time, he wants me to come to Charleston. I would never go just to meet Denny in Charleston, but Jay DeMarcus and Rascal Flatts is playing, and Jay is an old friend of ours and Jeff knows him from college. At the very beginning, when Denny and I were just friends, he was the road manager for Jay and Neal Coomer. Neal is so amazing, his voice would blow you away. He is so talented and great at everything he does. They were both in a band called East to West, and Georgia and I would go and see them all the time. All of us five became just the bestest of friends. I love Jay so much. I'm so hacky for him because Rascal Flatts is like the Beatles of country music! So Denny tells me that they're playing in Charleston, which is only two hours away from me, and I should come. It would be good for me. I'm going, "That sounds great." I'm just gonna see the band. Besides, the last time I saw Denny, I made it perfectly clear to him that I'm over him. I thought it was very sweet of him to ask 'cause he knows that I need to get away, he knows that I'm stressed.

I can see why Jeff and Georgia and everyone on my message boards say what they do about him (I know he kicked me to the curb and I promise you I do not forget that for one second!), but no matter what, Denny and I are really great friends and he knows what I need to lift me up again. He means well. He is worried about me, too, and he wants to do something. I know that there was no way that my friends were gonna let me go with him by myself—they think I'm all vulnerable right now, like I am not gonna be able to resist him. So I think I better ask him to get us all tickets so they are not hating his guts. Fingers crossed it all works out.

Back in the Groove

Denny did it! He called Jay, and got me, Jeff, Georgia, Jim, Ben, Zach, and Ben's friend Zach Ansley all tickets. He really came through; that's the good part of Denny. So not only did we get to see Jay perform this amazing concert, but we got to go backstage, too. I was so excited! It was the first time in so many weeks that I felt alive again. It felt great to be getting out of the house.

We had such a good time laughing and cutting up. After the show, we met the whole band and they were hugging me and Jay was telling me how great I looked. He said, "We don't consider you fat . . . just small challenged!" Well, that made me feel good! They were like my biggest cheerleaders, and it ended up to be the most perfect weekend ever. Denny was so sweet. He got me these pretty pink boxing gloves ('cause he knows I am such a girl!) and hot little jeans (which he says I am gonna fit into someday, but I just don't know if Bertha will make it!).

I am still hurting over Daddy, but I feel like I owe it to him—and to myself—to get back in the world and finish what I started. I got my food journal out and got myself back on Hourglass. I'm not ready to throw in the towel. There are too many adventures I have never gone on that I'm just waiting to have! Daddy was never a giver-upper . . . and I'm not one either!

Dear Daddy:

I miss you. Even though I know you're safe and in a great place, I miss you. I see your face, your beautiful eyes and your smile. I can feel your hands holding mine. I hear your laugh like you're right here beside me. I keep expecting to turn around and you'll be there. You are the greatest daddy, my hero, my knight in shining armor. If I am blessed enough, maybe I will one day find a man I can say this about again; I know you always wished this for me. But if I do not, please know that having a daddy like you was enough. Your love was enough for me. I never thought you'd leave me, and I never thought I would ever be without you. But we both had no control over this, and it can never change the way I feel about you.

Your presence will always be with me. Your face will haunt me, and my heart will never heal until I see you again. God created a masterpiece when he created my daddy and I was blessed to have you as my father for as long as I did.

I love you, Daddy . . . your baby, Ruby.

Another Family Crisis

My brother Clyde, Jim's daddy, had two strokes last night; he's a lot older than me. He has a heart of gold, and he would give you the shirt off his back. During Vietnam, he helped my mom take care of all of us. He got his GED, met and married Brenda, then fell at work and broke his hip. It took forever to heal. Then he was stepping out of our double wide trailer when he fell off the stairs. It was awful. His hip just popped out of his skin; he's not ever going to bend his left leg again and now his back's got a curve. My heart breaks for him; he's had his share of pain. He's fifty-six, and I worry so about him. He would have been dead if they hadn't gotten him to the hospital. They put him in ICU, so close after my father. The next thing I know, they say he's had a ministroke. He's on a blood thinner, and last night he had another stroke. He can't move his whole left side. My heart breaks for my mom, too. She's an angel. She's the strongest woman I know. There is no one else like her. She's the energizer of the whole family. She's always there for the ones she loves, no matter what. But no mother should have to watch her child suffer so. Especially not after so great a loss as seeing Daddy go. I wanna eat so badly. It's too close. I just lost my dad, and my brother and mother are hurtin' so bad now, too. I feel like everywhere I turn, there are obstacles being placed in my path. When I get worried about my family, I just can't focus on myself and it does make me wanna eat, eat, eat. It's an emotional reaction, I know. I recognize it, but that doesn't mean I can fight it. It feels selfish to think of myself when someone I love is suffering. I'm hoping for the best, for us all.

My Angel Boy

I am in awe of Jim sometimes. He always sees the good in things. Whether there are other kids around or he's playing games, this boy is incredible. People always ask, "Is he an angel?" because he is so nice; he never gets mad. He never overreacts. He's just so easygoing. Everyone is drawn to him. He's so polite and he respects people. He is the gentlest soul. But he made me so mad when he tried to get all tanned and he did it wrong. Well, you know, I had to go fix it for him. I had to take him back to the Tantastic tanning salon.

They are amazing and give the best tanning sprays, but I had to spray him myself to get it all just right. And Georgia and Jeff, they're all laughing at him and saying he looks like an Oompa-Loompa. Well, I just told them to hush up! I could see how good that tan made that boy feel about himself. And that's what matters. If you feel good about yourself, you don't gotta give a crapiola what anyone else thinks. I told him to hold his head up high. It's advice I give myself lots of times, too. It works. It really does.

From the Heart of Denny Starr

People always ask me how I met Ruby. It was through Jeff, actually. I went to Lee University in Tennessee with him. I remember he told me one day that a couple of his friends were coming to visit—Ruby and Georgia. And he warned me: "Now this Ruby, she is a big girl . . ." Well, the size didn't matter, because she and I hit it off so well. She was hilarious. I laughed and laughed and laughed. We were joined at the hip for that weekend, but after she left, we lost touch for a while. I was going on the road managing the band, but before I did, I went to a recording arts school in Ohio for six weeks. I don't remember why, but I decided to call Ruby. It was like we picked up exactly where we left off. I was on the road for two years and I called her all the time. I knew the weight was always something that held her back, and I tried to help her diet. I said, "I won't eat anything fried and I won't eat any red meat"—which when you're on the road is impossible, because it's all burgers and fries! But I wanted to help her.

I also wanted to be with her. I would go to Savannah and stay with her when I had a break, and she and Georgia would go to our shows. When I first started to get to know her, she had these pictures of supermodels and TV stars on her walls—she loved Beverly Hills, 90210, and I had to watch it with her religiously. She admired beauty. And she was beautiful herself. Even at her size, she was not going anywhere if her makeup or her hair wasn't just right.

Jeff had already moved to L.A., and we both loved L.A., so I suggested we move out there together. That started that—we were out there for eight years. But we had gotten real close even before then. She was my best friend. We were just so compatible, and we could tell each other anything. We had so much in common—we even liked the same music. At the time, we were into the Doors and the Eagles and Fleetwood Mac and we used to crank up the music and dance. It felt right. We were really good together. We even talked about getting married, but the physical just wasn't there. It was the weight that came between us. I couldn't get past it.

I have known Ruby on lots of diets before, but this time, I do think she's going to do it. I know how hard it is. But now with so many people watching and so many people supporting her, this is it. Sometimes she gets worried and scared. I tell her, "You will do it. It doesn't matter how fast, just as long as you never quit."

And in my opinion, she doesn't have to be 150 pounds; I think she could be 200 or 250 and that would be okay. I think she will get down to a regular size. In the past, she was always overwhelmed at the end goal, how far away it was. But now it's so close. She sees it in her reach, and she sees what an inspiration she is and how she's changing lives. That's something we always believed would happen.

I know she wants badly to figure out how she got this way. We talked about it one time, and she started crying. She grew up on military bases, trailer parks . . . it could have been something that scared her as a child while she was walking down the street. But I know what she fears. She fears someone hurt her or abused her.

I also think she was scared all this time of what would happen if she lost the weight. The weight is who she was; this big girl with so much personality. If she loses it, then who would she be? But I think she knows now that it's just a shell, not the person inside. That will never change.

People have always wondered or questioned me, "You're a good-looking guy, a personal trainer, around all these pretty girls . . . why Ruby?" That's easy: you have never met anybody who loves you like she does, the way she does, with all her heart. Her heart is the biggest thing about her. I can truthfully say no one has ever loved me that much . . . and probably no one ever will.

—Denny

Ruby's Smile

Denny is such a great songwriter! He wrote the lyrics to this song just for me, while his writing partner Mark Kauffman wrote the beautiful music. It's called "Smile (Ruby's Song)," and it makes me smile and cry at the same time. I was so moved, I wanted to share the lyrics with everyone:

"Smile (Ruby's Song)"
lyrics by Denny Starr, music by Mark Kauffman

One smile from her can set you free
Her life is like a tapestry
Painted on a wall for ones she loves

She'll hold your hand right till the end
She's everybody's closest friend
Now it's her own race she has to run

(chorus)
So now it's time to be the one in front
Let everybody see just how much you love
And let the love that they send back to you
Be the hand you hold as you make this dream
come true

'Cause everybody loves to see you smile
As these days pass by will still be here
Keeping faith to face our fears
And know for sure that we've already won

Because we've loved and laughed and cried
The memories we'll hold inside
And make new ones with every rising sun

And now it's time to be the one in front
Let everybody see just how much you love
And let the love that they send back to you
Be the hand you hold as you make this dream
come true
'Cause everybody loves to see you smile

Ride Ruby ride
Let your beautiful eyes be our guide
Ride Ruby ride
(repeat chorus)

8   TIRED OF WEIGHTING

L.A. or Bust

I'm in L.A. on vacation, but I left my Hourglass meals at home. I think I have everything under control. I know what I can and can't eat, and I'm gonna pay real close attention to what I put in my mouth. Really I am. Anyway, I'm having a blast! It is so much fun being back. Living here for a while was great—I still have so many friends I want to meet up with and places I want to visit again. I can't wait to see my Formosa kids (who are definitely not kids anymore!): Irina, Katcha, Anna, and Tomas. I can't wait to see Marcia, Michael and Melissa and their new baby, Parker; and Cynthia and Cole's new baby; and Ryland, too! I can't wait to see Brittany and I especially can't wait for us all to hang out together and catch up! I always wish I had more time to spend with them. But I feel good. I feel happy and relaxed. I'm headed to the beach now for a walk. Talk to you later!

Where Did I Go Wrong?

I'm home now and not a hacky camper. I stepped on the scale today, and I gained three pounds. I wasted freakin' two weeks—I could have been ten pounds smaller! What happened? I am so upset and angry. I am going to freakin' figure it out, because I cannot waste any more time.

My nutritionist told me to write everything down in a food journal. Well, I did this the whole time I was on vacation, just like she said. I keep going over it and over it. I don't think I ate that much: a banana here, fresh fruit, a protein bar, two pita chips, some hummus . . . After dinner at night, I ate some low-fat Cool Whip with blueberries. What's wrong with that? It is really not a lot of food. So what happened? I am scared, really scared. This is the place I have been at so many times before when I just toss it all and give up. I am buggin'! And we are throwing Georgia this Hacky Wacky fortieth b-day party and Danna is comin' in and all I can think is, "Ruby, you failed again." I need to get help. I need to ask my team what I did to cause this. They are going to be so disappointed in me. I am really dreading having to tell them . . .

Reading the Writing on the Label

Well, I did it. I told my nutritionist Helen first. I told her, "I didn't hardly eat anything." But I don't think she believes me. The pounds just didn't come out of thin air. I did something to put them back on. So we went through my journal. I showed her how good I had been, and she kept shaking her head like, "No, no, no . . ." I feel so stupid! She told me I have been eating the wrong protein bars. I gotta look at the sugar, the protein, the fat. She said some of those bars are not snacks; they're supposed to be eaten instead of a meal. Are you kidding me? I was eating them *in addition to* my three meals. In my mind, a protein bar is diet food. Any protein bar. Now I gotta be reading every wrapper to see if they're good ones or bad ones? Well, that is just too much! She said that I can't just eat all the nutritious food I want, all the health bars, all the fruit and oatmeal, and still expect to lose weight. Well, then what's the point? Why don't I just grab a Milky Way, then? This is *soooo* frustrating.

I saw my trainer Reese next so I could tell him how upset I am. I thought maybe he'd have some ideas. Reese got right to the point: he wanted to know if I exercised on vacation. Well, of course I did! I was real good. I did a ton of walking when we were sightseeing. I made sure I always walked everywhere. There was no hopping in a taxi or a car. "Did you sweat?" he asked me. Well, L.A. is just not as hot as Savannah, so no, I didn't hardly sweat any at all. Reese said that means the intensity of my exercise wasn't there; if I didn't break a sweat, the workout just plain wasn't working. And he can tell, because today I was all huffing and puffing and I could barely get through my time on the treadmill. So now I am backward on my workout, too. I was dying today! I'm confused and disappointed; I feel like I am back where I started. The scary thing is, I felt like I was doing so good; like maybe I had this thing finally beat. But I didn't. I messed it all up.

Birthday Party Blues

Jeff is trying to do Georgia's party planning by himself—he says he doesn't want to distract me from my diet and that makes me mad. I want to be happy, I want to be making this the best party for Georgia ever. But right now, I feel totally alone. No one really understands how hard this is. I am not in a good place, and I cannot hide it. My friends and family are here to support me, but I have to take this journey by myself. It's Ruby's road, no one else's.

Anyway, I was happy to see Danna today. I miss her so bad. We have known each other since we were teenagers and we have always kept in touch. I just hugged her and hugged her. She says I look great; she can see the transformation. Well, I can't. I guess I am just in a foul mood. I don't wanna ruin her visit for everyone, but I can't get those three freakin' pounds outta my head!

Every time Danna was back in town before, we would go out to eat. But this time, I had to take my preplanned meal with me. It's great hanging out with her, but I miss piggin' out like we used to. My girls were trying their best to cheer me up. We were getting ready for the party, and they're showing me all these pretty dresses and I got to pick the ones they were wearing. I love to see my friends all dressed up; I love that they can wear whatever they want. But sometimes I wish I could, too. I am wearing this shirt. It is not an outfit. It's just a big ol' shirt. I can't wait for the day that I can pick out an outfit to wear to go dancing or to a party. Danna looks so beautiful in everything she wears because she only weighs like a hundred pounds. Will I ever get there?

Georgia loved her party and everyone had a great time. Me, too, even despite my setback. I used to love going to parties and pigging out with my friends. When I can't and everyone else can, it makes me feel like, even in a room full of people, I am totally alone in this. I am there with my preplanned meal. I can smell it in the microwave and I am so freakin' annoyed. Well, y'all go ahead! There is food everywhere; just dig in! They had hot dogs, hamburgers, and chips. For a little while there, I was not a hacky camper. I wanted to eat what they were eating bad, and I wanted to join in the fun and I couldn't. I wanted not to have to think about my weight or my diet; I wanted to just feel free and have fun like everyone else. Over-all, it was a great day, but the whole food thing made it hard for me, very hard. After the party I was even more upset about my weight gain and I wanted to get to the bottom of it.

I sat down with Dr. Brewerton; I really wanted to see things clearer. I told him I went off my plan. I thought I could do it on my own; I thought I was doing a good job and making smart choices. I didn't eat candy or pizza. When I was done talking, he said, "Ruby, you are going to have difficulty doing it on your own. You can't go off your plan." He said I've assembled this great team of experts, and that I'm afraid to trust my team. Then he said he's worried I won't reach my goal. He's worried about how I've handled this situation and what I've done. Then he added if this is my choice, if this is how I am going to do things, then I am going to fail.

That's it? It's over? I am going to fail because I didn't eat my preplanned meal on vacation? Well, here comes the Kleenex! I just cried and cried, not because I was hurting that he told me I would fail, but because what he said really made sense. He said I don't trust. I didn't see it that way at all. I just saw me trying to stick to my diet. But he says I have to trust; I have to surrender to folks who know better, who know how to help me. I have done this on my own forever, but I do not know best. That was an awakening for me. I guess I have always had a hard time trusting people. It's very freakin' hard for me to trust. But Dr. Brewerton says if I continue to fight these battles on my own, I am never gonna win. I am gonna have to let go. I am gonna have to have faith that all these people who are helping me, that their way is the right way. He doesn't want me to make all the choices myself, because whenever I do, I put on those three pounds or thirty or three hundred. I left there trying to take in everything he said.

Whenever I feel shaken, whenever I am losing faith, I have to reach out to God. So I took Georgia, Danna, Jeff, Jim, Ben, and Zach to the church where we met as kids. It's the one place I have always felt safe. Pastor McDaniel called me up and he prayed for me. At first, I was "nerdous" being up in front of everyone. It's not like being on TV when you're up front in church. There you're standing, in front of God, and He is a much tougher audience. The whole church was behind me and I could hear them praying. I started to feel it. I started to feel myself standing a little taller. Knowing that people are out there for me, rooting for me, praying for me, it just gave me the most unbelievable strength. It's really important to me that God is gonna help me with this. He helped me get started, but I need more help. I see that now. I am trying to put my faith and trust in my team; I have got an army behind me! And I'm going to use all their power and knowledge as best as I can.

FROM THE HEART OF JIM GETTINGER

I have so many favorite Ruby moments—it's hard to just narrow it down to one. But if I had to choose one that's her all-time craziest? Well, there's the time she tells me, "I wanna cut your hair, Jim. You know I can do it. You know you can trust me . . ." I am looking at her, going, "Ruby, what do you know about cutting hair?" She gives me that big smile and says, "Oh, I know lots. I have watched plenty of people do it." Watched? Have you ever picked up a pair of scissors? I knew I was in trouble, but she keeps telling me, "I promise you it's gonna look good. Trust me!"

You just can't say no to Ruby. She doesn't take no for an answer.
EVER! So she cuts it all right: she puts a colander on top of my
head and cuts my hair around the edges. This, she says, is how
you shape it. Then she puts my hair in ponytails and she trims the
ponytails. When she puts them down, one side of my hair is way
above my ears and the other is hangin' over them. Well, of course
we had to call a friend who cuts hair professionally to fix me
because my hair was such a wreck after being Ruby-fied! But she
means well, I know that, and we had a good laugh over it. That's
just Ruby. She thinks that she can do anything. She lets nothing
stand in her way. She has never let her weight control her life.
She went out; she had fun with her friends—even at her biggest.
She didn't let life pass her by. She inspires us all . . . even if she
is never getting a job any day soon as a hairstylist! If you see her
comin' at you with a comb and scissors . . . run!

—Jim

9   MAKING WAVES

Best Lifeguards Ever

I know I can float in the water. As long as my tippy toes can touch the bottom of the pool, I am not too worried. But I have never been able to swim. I just never learned. I was doing this water aerobics class with Jeff, Danna, and Georgia today, and they were telling me, "Ruby, just try it. You can do it. You can swim across the pool." There was this swim instructor, Amy Bradley, and she showed me how to do this little doggie paddle and I was saying, "Y'all, I am going to drown!" But everyone was rooting me on: "Just do it. You won't go under; you're gonna stay up." Yeah, right. So I started in the shallow end, and I felt pretty silly and nerdous. The side of the pool that I can grab onto looks a mile away. And the whole time, I'm wondering, if I go under, is someone gonna be strong enough to pull me out? There's no life preserver that's gonna fit over me, y'all. What are you thinking?

I know what I'm thinking: "God help me!" But I wanted to do this. I wanted to conquer this. I knew that if I could do just this one little thing, I could do so much more. I took a deep breath and off I went, doing the doggie paddle! I was getting closer and closer, and more and more tired, but I couldn't stop, because if I did, I would sink like a stone. Well, I made it. I swam across that big, deep pool. Everyone was cheering for me and I felt *so good*. I swam, y'all! I did it! And I learned something, too; sometimes I just have to believe these people. They care about me and wanna help. When they tell me to trust, they mean it. The way I see it, I have a choice: I can sink or I can swim. And I'm swimming now.

The Big Fight

Today was weigh-in. I wanted to drop ten more pounds since the last time I weighed-in, but I only lost seven. I know I should be happy with any loss, but I've been pushing myself so hard. I wanted to cry, but I didn't want my trainer, Reese, to see me do that, so I just got real quiet. He could see it in my face and he was trying to cheer me on, but I can't pretend I'm happy when I'm not. That scale sometimes is my worst enemy, because what it says really affects how I feel. If it's a good number—more than I thought—then I am on cloud nine. If it's less or if the scale stood still, I'm miserable. Even worse—if I've gone up—it can just ruin my whole mood for a week. I am working so freakin' hard I want the scale to show exactly how hard.

On top of that, Reese told me he has concerns about my meal plan. He wants me to put some whole foods—fruits, vegetables and meats—into my diet. He thinks it has too much fat and salt and processed stuff. He said everyone is holding my hand and that these prepackaged meals are what he calls a "quick fix." He also thinks that there's nothing quick about them, because my weight is taking so long to come off!

When I told Dr. Bradley and Dr. Brewerton, they were like, "Nuh-uh, Ruby. You need to stay on the plan. You cannot go this alone." Then they brought up L.A. again: "Look at what happened when you tried to do this by yourself. You are not there yet." Well, that made me feel a little like a baby, or like I'm not smart enough to take care of myself. But I have to trust that these experts know what they're doing. It's pretty easy to see: When I am on my prepackaged meal program, I lose weight. When I am not, I gain. So there you go. But they were all fighting about it. And honestly, I wished I could have just stayed out of it! I don't like anyone's feelings to get hurt. I don't wanna pick sides. What do I do? Who do I listen to? I hate when people aren't getting along. So I called a meeting with all of them. I said, "I need y'all to get together and agree on something because I am confused. I am getting mixed messages. I need one plan." Well, they took me up on it and they're having a meeting. I'm scared! I don't want them mad at each other. I see the fire in Reese's eyes . . . this is gonna be uggy.

Truce

Well, we had our "summit" today, as Dr. Brewerton calls it. We all met up at Magnolia House. He's like the referee between everyone. He tells me, "Be ruthlessly honest, Ruby. Don't worry about hurting people's feelings." I just sat there, mostly listening, and the tempers were flowing; everyone's got a lot of different opinions and they were not afraid to speak them. I could see the tension on their faces. Then they started talking over each other, and it got louder and louder. I was feeling scared. So Dr. Brewerton made me leave the room. They sent me out of my *own* meeting! I didn't like that at all! I should have been there. It was about *me*. I chose every one of them. It was all very strange. I hoped they weren't gonna be mean to each other. I never wanted it to come to this, "Who's right? Who's wrong?"

They were in there a long time and I could hear them yelling at each other through the door. I was thinking, "Oh no. This is all my fault." I really didn't expect them to come to an agreement. I began sweatin' more than when I'm doing one of Reese's workouts. Then it got real quiet and they asked me to come back in. They were all smiles. There was peace! They all agreed that I should stick with the meal program. I said that's fine; I haven't cheated, but they told me I was BS-ing them! Sometimes I do not like the way Dr. B. comes across. He may not mean to, but he can sound rude and controlling, and that approach will definitely not work with me! That really bugged me. I may be a lot of things, but I am not a BS-er! I said to them that a BS-er is someone who knows what they are doing. They preplan. But if I do *not* know what I am doing, then you cannot accuse me of BS-ing. I am on a journey to learn and find out things I didn't know before, so let's be careful with our words. I felt a little beaten up, but after six months, I know they really care—they are not only doing their jobs, they are being good friends, too. And if they get passionate about this stuff, it's because they truly want me to succeed.

Finally Out of the Fours

Jeff and Jim hid my scale! I looked all over the house and I couldn't find it. I'm looking under Jeff's bed, in his closets, under his mess of clothes. It's nowhere. They didn't want me to weigh in, because they know that if it doesn't say I weigh under 400, I am gonna be so upset with myself. I am supposed to wait two weeks to weigh in, but I want to do it every day. I just can't wait. So they think they're protecting me, but they're just making me mad! Finally Jeff pulled the scale out of the broiler in the oven! Is he crazy? That is just uggy—not to mention it could have caused a fire! So I stepped on it and the voice—it has the pretty little lady voice—goes, "Hello. I'm ready . . . " Well, I'm not! I hold my breath every single time I step on that thing. And it says, "394.2 pounds." I wanna throw a party! I can be done with the fours now, I am in the threes. I know I have a long way to go—another 250 pounds—but it feels so good. Dr. Bradley keeps reminding me to take it slow; not to push myself too much, because we want the weight not just to come off but to stay off. I understand where he's coming from. But I am just so hacky when I see those numbers dropping! I would do anything to make them come down faster!

FROM THE HEART OF GEORGIA'S SONS, BEN AND ZACH THOMPSON

I love that Ruby pushes other people—to reach for the stars and achieve their dreams. You see her doing it for herself, but she does it for everyone else, too. Music is what I am most passionate about, and Ruby sees that. So she does everything she can to help me with it. She gave me my first guitar when I was about twelve. I was overtaken by it, but I didn't know how to go about learning how to play. So Ruby, being the loving aunt that she is, threatened to sell it on eBay if I didn't pick it up right then and there. She said I had no choice; I had to learn right away! Who does that? But I am so glad she did, because she gave me the motivation I needed to start playing and I have been hooked ever since.

One of my favorite musicians of all time is John Mayer. If it were up to Ruby she'd find a way to meet him and tell him so. She always says, "Believe it and it will happen." She is so determined about things and thinks everyone else should be, too. Will I meet John? As I've learned from Ruby, it's not so much an "if" for me as it is a "when." Especially if she has anything to do with it. She is like a second mom to me; she raised me with my own mother since birth. I can tell her anything. When we first started doing the TV show, it was surreal. Then it aired and people started stopping her on the street That's how I knew something big was happening. People travel thousands of miles just to see her. Everyone who meets Ruby loves her. But I'm lucky enough to have her in my life forever.

—Ben

Ruby has been a second mother to me. She is always kind, caring, and takes the time to listen to whatever I have to say. I remember when she was living in L.A., my mom, brother, and I really missed having her in our lives every day. So when went to see her in the summer, she threw us all a great big birthday party, to celebrate all the birthdays she'd missed while she was away. She always knows how to make people feel special and appreciated. It's what I love about her most.

—Zach

10 FREEDOM

Baby, I Can Drive My Car!

I haven't driven in six years because I couldn't fit in a car. I couldn't even get my leg under the steering wheel. I never ever wore a seat belt either—because it wouldn't go more than halfway across me. I had to fake it so I wouldn't get a ticket! (I know how bad that is. I really do.) I was always relying on other people to drive me here or there. I felt like a baby; I had to ask everyone to just get from one place to the next. But today was different! I got in the car with Jim and off we went. I was free! I didn't have to depend on anyone. Jim was a little scared . . . he was like, "You sure you remember how to do this?" I didn't have a license that was valid anymore, so Jeff was all over me to take a "refresher course." What was I supposed to do? Go to the Department of Motor Vehicles and say, "I haven't driven in six years 'cause I was too fat?!" I had lied about my weight on the original license. (All women lie about their weight. All men do, too—they just don't admit it.) But Jeff convinced me to get a new license by telling me I could put my new weight on it—and that made me happy. I look huge in that old picture! I was like five hundred pounds. He's just worried about me, because if I was to get into an accident, the paramedics or the doctors at the hospital couldn't work on me like they do most other people. I guess I worry about that, too.

Road Rage

I took my driving test today—I wanted to kill Jeff. The lady administering the test was so strict. She told me I have to slam on the brakes and parallel park while Jeff is in the backseat making me laugh the whole time. I just couldn't concentrate. Then she made me drive around a bunch of cones to show how good I could steer. Well, why would I ever drive around cones in real life? I was knockin' so many of them down, but it's 'cause I couldn't see what I was doing. I'm too big to turn around and check behind me. I hit four of them— maybe more. But she passed me anyway. Barely. And I got a new license with a beautiful new picture. Jeff got me some seat belt extenders so I can wear a seat belt now. I know it's safer, but I hate it because it chokes me. I also think it makes me look fatter—wrinkling my shirt and all. And it feels like a girdle! But I'll buckle up anyway if it makes him happy.

Just Say No

Jim made me drive him to Bojangles' today because he was hungry. I get to go outside driving for the first time, and here I am in a fast-food drive-thru! The whole time, I am thinking about my past, how I used to live in these fast-food places. Jim can't even make up his mind about what he wants. He's making me sit there at the drive-thru window, looking at the pictures and smelling sweet potato pie and buttermilk biscuits, while he decides. That is so cruel! It's like waving my favorite foods in my face and singin', "You can't have any!" Finally—it felt like hours—he ordered a Cajun filet sandwich with french fries and a sweet tea. He had to go and order the sweet tea, as if those tempting fries weren't enough to drive me crazy. The old Ruby would have eaten something really big and bad, and that would have been it; it would've blown my diet for two years. I swear I could have slapped Jim! But then I told myself to simmer down. He should be able to eat what he wants to eat. This is a demon that I have to conquer. Not him. I had to sit in the car and smell that food and it was killin' me. But I did it. I resisted. I didn't eat any. Not even one fry. Take *that* chicken biscuit. Ruby don't need you no more.

The Finish Line

I walked a mile today. I needed to prove to myself—and my team—that I could. For most people, this is no big deal. But for me, it's a major milestone. There was a time, not too long ago, when I could barely walk a block without feeling out of breath. I wanted to do this. I needed to do this. So I went with Jeff to my favorite park. I told him, "I gotta walk it fast. I gotta get it over with; the sooner the better." When I started, I had no idea how far it was. A mile doesn't sound like that much, but it is. It's an eternity! I was like, "Jeff, I am not gonna be able to make it." He just kept on talking because *I* couldn't. I couldn't breathe. I kept my eyes on the ground because if I looked up and I saw how much farther I had to go, I would have given up right then and there. I could feel my legs burning—they have never felt so heavy. I was thinking, "Lord, I am gonna die!" It was killing me. We got halfway there and I was thinking my knees were gonna buckle under me. Then we made this turn and I could see the finish line. I was so hot I thought it might be a mirage. My legs felt like they weighed two hundred pounds more than usual. But I kept on getting closer and closer, walking faster and faster, just thinking, "You're almost there, You're almost there." Then Jeff said to me, "Rube. You did it." I had chills all over me. I was all cold and sweaty and shaking. It was the most awesome feeling ever, to conquer this. I cried because, as I like to say, "It was

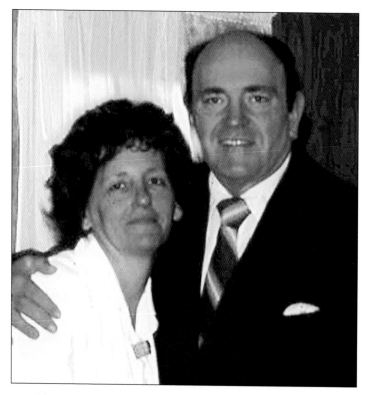

I have a wonderful family. This is my daddy, James Edward Gettinger, and my mom, Ann Gettinger.

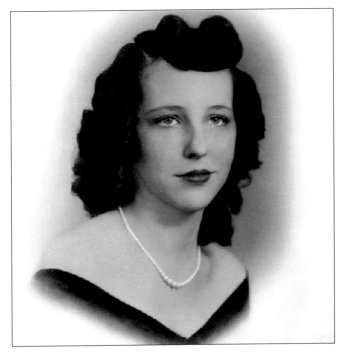

I love this picture of my mom in her younger days—she is
the light of my life . . .

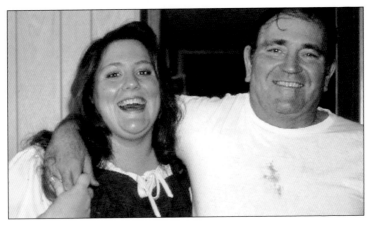

And I especially like this one of me and my dad. Ever since
he passed, I miss him so much.

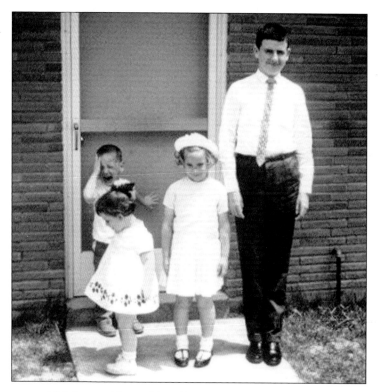

This is me with my older siblings, Clyde, Jamie, and John,
after I thumped John over the head with a Bible.
Who does that?

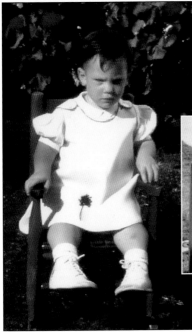

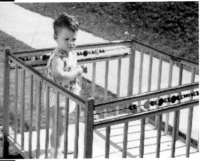

I still don't look like much of a "hacky camper" in these pictures . . .

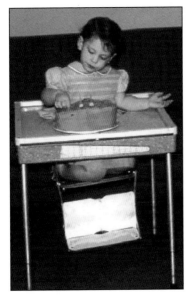

but I seem to be in a much better mood here. Who doesn't love birthday cake?!

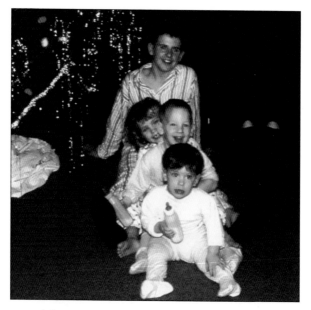

This is me again with John, Jamie, and Clyde
on Christmas morning . . .

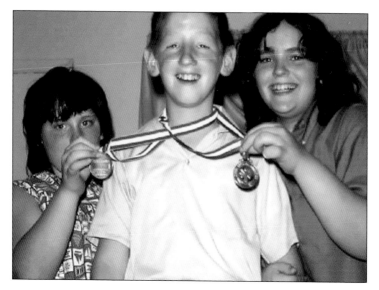

and years later on the day
John won the races at the Special Olympics.

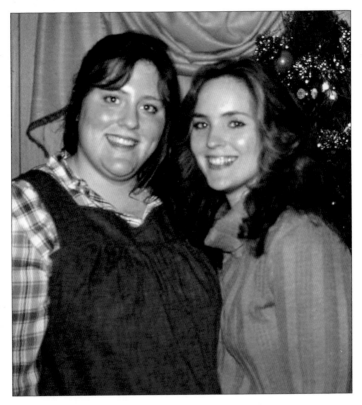

And here's me and Jamie as teenagers. She's been so great,
helping me recover my childhood memories by collecting as
many photos of us when we were little kids as she can!

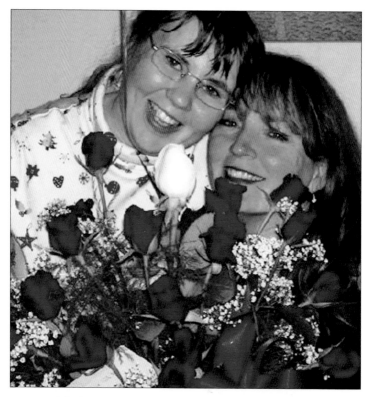

That's Jamie again with my adorable niece Karen . . .

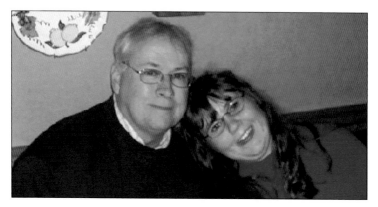

And here's Karen with my wonderful brother-in-law Steve.
They've all been so supportive of me!

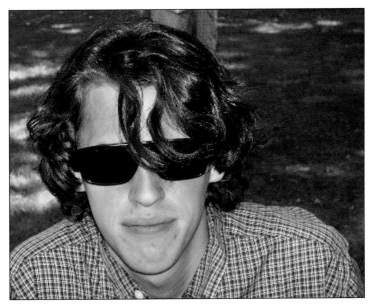

And who doesn't recognize my fabulous nephew Jim
from the show? (Even with his sunglasses on!)

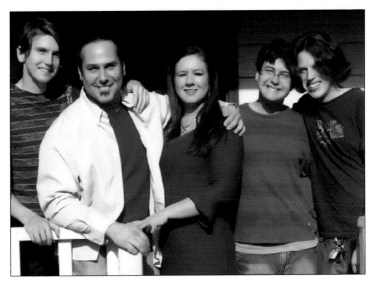

Here's Jim again with the whole gang—Ben, Jeff, Georgia,
and Zach. I love them all so much and am grateful to them
for taking this journey with me!

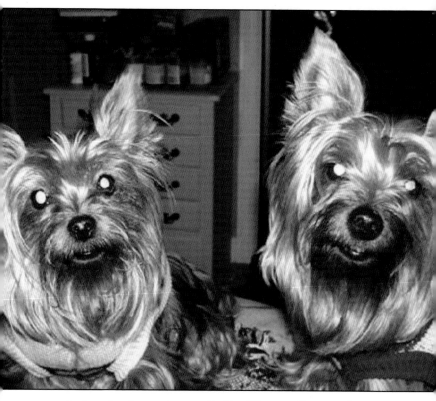

And you just have to love my "babies," Foxy and Lucy, too!
Aren't they cute?

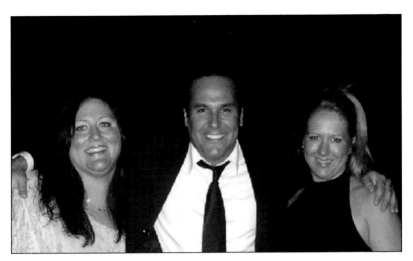

Here I am with besties Jeff and Georgia.
I'm so blessed to have such a big family of lifelong
and fun-loving friends, including . . .

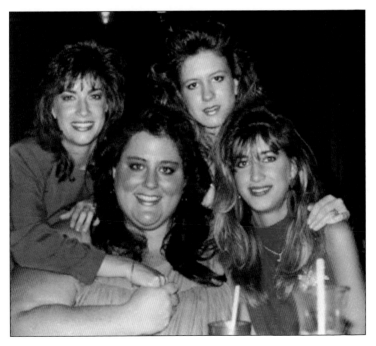

Chris, Danna, and Georgia . . .

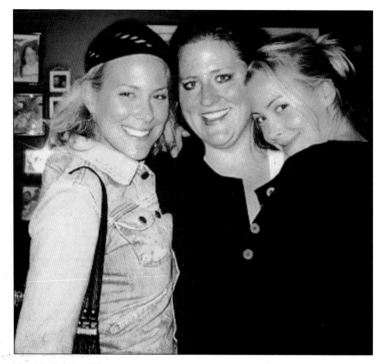

Brittany and Cynthia . . .

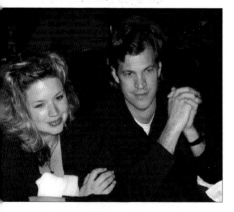

Leslie and Greg . . .

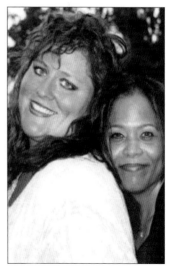

Marcia . . .

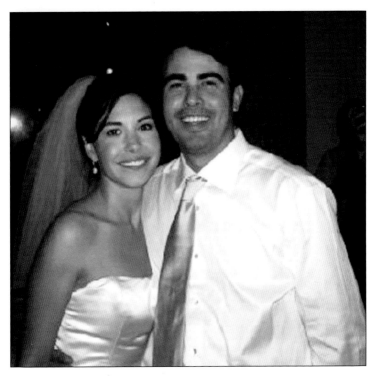

Melissa and Michael . . .

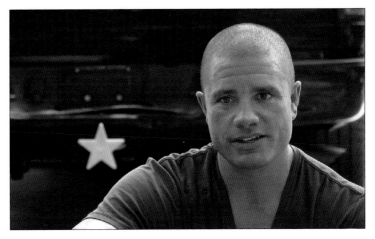

and Denny, too.

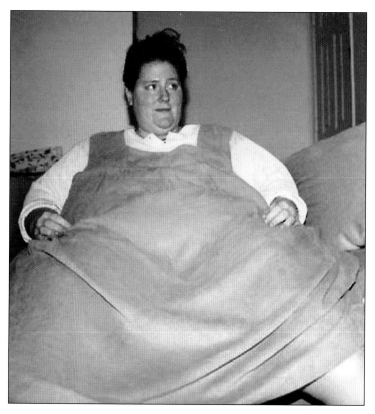

Here I am at my heaviest—weighing 716 pounds . . .

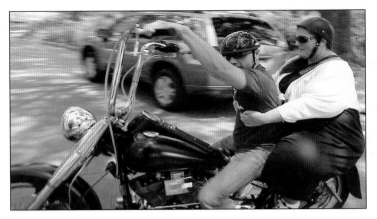

having the time of my life riding motorcycles . . .

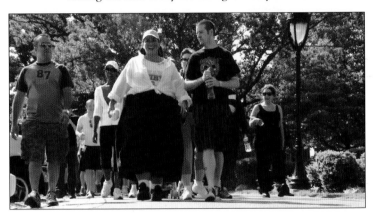

walking in as many cities as I can get to . . .

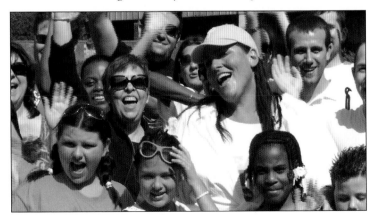

meeting new people . . .

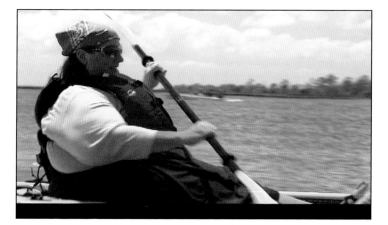

kayaking . . .

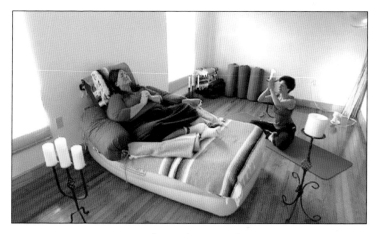

and even doing yoga!

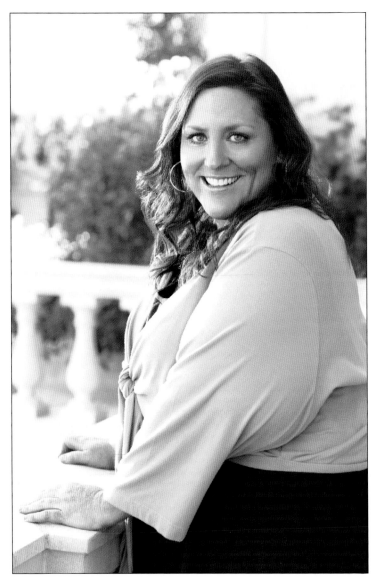

And although this is where the photos end,
it's not where the story ends. This is me at
333 pounds and still pursuing my goals.

sensitivity to me." I walked a mile in fifteen minutes! I want so bad to be a winner, and I was a winner today. I told Jeff he better go braggin' to everyone for me. And I'm pretty sure he did. Jeff is my man friend and soul mate. I love him so much! The woman who gets him will be the most blessed woman ever. Not only is Jeff a hottie, but he is a true-blue southern gentleman. He opens doors for me and I'm not even his girlfriend! Jeff can make me laugh like no other and he is a manly man, too. He loves his doggie, Mellie, just like I love my doggies. We're alike in that way; we both love our animals and *all* animals in general. And Jeff has been through a lot. He lost his niece Morgan Parsons when she was only eighteen and then a year later he lost his nephew Caleb, who was only two. Caleb was like a son to Jeff. But no matter what Jeff goes through, he never loses his faith in God. He still finds a way to laugh and be thankful. He is truly an inspiration to me! And I'm glad he was there for me today and every day.

From the Heart of Jeff Parsons

I first met Ruby at the skating rink. We were probably about thirteen or fourteen at the time. Me and my friend asked if we could push her around the ice—we didn't ask in a mean way. She was kinda skating around slow, and we said, "Do you want us to push you?" And she was like, "Yeah." Not embarrassed at all, mind you! So we did. It was less work for her after all. We became friends that day. Isn't that crazy? She ended up joining our church youth group and choir and I introduced her and Georgia.

That was right when Georgia and I started liking each other. As soon as we were old enough to drive, it was automatic hanging out. The three of us were inseparable. And Ruby had lots of guy friends. She didn't have a problem whatsoever making friends. She had and still has this infectious joy, this way of making you forget her size. You just get caught up in her personality and her faith, and you don't see the rest. It disappears. She has this strong personality—she will tell you what she thinks and what she feels—but at the same time, there's this childlike innocence to her. It's almost like she goes through life thinking, "I'm having fun. What is wrong with y'all?" She's fearless like a toddler—like she's gonna laugh right off a cliff!

The plan was never that we would be permanent roommates. I moved in with her because I was going to find a fixer house. I found one the second year I was here, but at that point, it was like old times. I didn't want to leave; she didn't want me to go. But we're truly the odd couple. I'm messy and she's a neat freak. I drive her crazy. She literally will find toothpaste that I didn't run down the drain and start yelling at me: "That is nasty, Jeff! That is disgusting! Who wants to see your spit?" The only reason we've lasted this long is we care enough about each other not to sweat the small stuff. Toothpaste—or piles of my clothes on the floor—will never come between us.

When the producers asked me and Georgia and Jim to be a part of this show, none of us was thinking this would be hard or invasive or that it would take long hours. We were only thinking of Ruby. She has loved harder than anyone I know. She deserves this. Every time I get a little weary, I have to switch my mind to what it's doing for her. She wants her truth to be out there, and we're helping her do it. Even if I am tired of the cameras in our lives, I do it for her. Anyone who knows her would feel the same way—you'd climb mountains if she asked you to. She just has this magnetic personality. You are drawn to her. I have been walking down the street with her recently when she's been mobbed by people who wanted to meet her, touch her, share their stories, tell her how she has inspired them. I get thousands of e-mails literally, from people asking me, "Jeff, please have Ruby call me . . ." We are mobbed with people no matter where we go. She has literally stopped traffic because someone wants to jump out of a car and talk to her. It's thrilling for me—for all of her friends really—because the whole world is finally getting to know what I have always known: what an amazing human being Ruby Gettinger is.

—Jeff

11   EXTRA SUPPORT

That Don't Come in My Size

When I look at myself in the mirror, I still see a fat girl. I don't see what I've lost—just what I have left to lose. I don't see what other people see. They tell me, "It is such a major difference!" but I look at myself from every angle, and I swear, I don't see much of a change at all. When I called Brittany and told her about me losing ninety pounds, she wanted to come out and see for herself. She says I am a Skinny Minnie now, which is so sweet. She wanted to give me a whole new look and take me shopping. I appreciate it, truly, but shopping is not exactly fun for me. It is so hard to find anything but old-lady clothes. Big-ladies clothes are just meant to cover you up; they're not fashionable, they're not sexy. They don't flatter anyone. They just kinda hang there over you like a tent.

It's like you go up to a certain weight and they punish you by making you wear this stuff. Like they're saying, "Shame on y'all for being this big! You are now going to wear uggy clothes!" But Brittany was determined that she was going to give me a makeover. So I said okay. I didn't want to go into the big-girl stores because I was proud that I was ninety pounds lighter and I thought surely by now something "normal size" might fit me. But nothing in there fit me at all. Not one piece of clothing. There was this one shirt that I thought looked big enough, but I could barely get my arm through it. It just wouldn't stretch more than halfway around me. There was nothin' for me there, and I was getting down. I was looking at myself thinking, "Ninety freakin' pounds and you still can't get any decent clothes." I am so tired of always lookin' and never finding. So to be sweet—and I guess to not make the day a total waste—Brit got me a stylish little hat. I love it! Thank God for accessories.

Right after our little disappointing "shopping spree," I swore to myself I'd start a support group for women who are size twelve, fourteen, and up . . . I know what they're going through and they know what I'm going through, so, "Why," I thought, "shouldn't we all get together and help each other out?" I am gonna call it Fat Night! Jeff thinks that it's a bad idea to call it that; people are gonna be all sensitive over the word *fat*. But like I said, I am honest about my situation. Fat is fat. There is no other word for it! And to me fat has had a bad name for too long. The truth is, fat people are beautiful people, too! So why not start changing that word for the positive! So I started calling everyone I knew who might wanna join. I have a lot of fat friends, but I am the fattest in the group, so they shouldn't feel bad about being part of it all. The name of the club didn't seem to matter to any of them: They were all so excited! This was the first time I ever put anything together to help people who are struggling with obesity. We all had a great time. Every single woman at my meeting is totally beautiful, and they have every right to feel beautiful. But designers have forgotten about the big girls. We're not all that different. We still want things that are pretty. Things that let us feel like we're in the land of the living! We want to hold our heads up, too.

Dr. Bradley has a friend, Anthony, who is the chair of the fashion department of the Savannah College of Art and Design (go figure that!), so he called him for me and he asked him if maybe he and his students could make me some pretty clothes. I was praying that this guy would say yes and he did. He's gonna make me something beautiful. But I was so nerdous to meet him and his class. Having my best friends, Georgia and Leslie, with me made it a lot easier. I was sure he had never fit anyone with this body! I told them I wanted something cute for once, to feel better about myself. They asked me all sorts of questions like "What look do you like?" I said cowboy boots and sundresses. And the hippie look! I'd love to be a hippie! I have never been able to find any flowy skirts in flowery, bright, hippie-style fabrics that come in my size. I loved Anthony's ideas and the fabrics were just breathtaking— all sorts of bright colors that felt so soft and sheer and silky.

He wanted to spotlight my upper body—do something real sexy—and hide Bertha. I am all for that! I feel like a movie star. I get my own designers! I get people making clothes just for me that will fit! There is such love here . . . these are the first people who have ever listened to what I want. I am a very happy hippie just thinking about it. I can't wait to see what they come up with.

Me on the Runway

It's been three weeks since I met with the design students Dr. Bradley set me up with. Today they had me come in for a fashion show. I did the runway twirl! They made me all these beautiful clothes in flowy fabrics and beautiful colors and patterns. I loved it! I was looking through these racks of outfits and I came to the pants. I'm like, "Are you out of your minds? Leggings? I have not worn pants in thirty years!" And you know, I can be a stubborn mule sometimes. I was insisting it would not go over my leg and Anthony kept pushing me to go and try them on. A lot of people make mistakes; they all said, "It'll fit, Ruby." But I have lived in this body. I know what will fit and what won't. Well, Anthony kept insisting, and all these kids who made them for me are sitting there giving me the guilt trip. So I finally went in back to put them on—just to prove them wrong.

Well, was I in for a surprise. They *did* fit; they were actually too big. It felt so weird to see my foot and my ankle coming out of a pair of pants. I was just having so much fun! For the first time, I felt like I was in style, I was in fashion. They made my dream come true. They made me feel like a sexy woman! And I think those students learned something: it doesn't matter if you're designing for a size 6 or size 8X. I looked at those kids: these are the world's future designers. I want them all to remember me. I'm gonna remember them. I hope they're inspired. Because if they made me this happy, think of how many other people they could make happy. How many dreams they could make come true. Anthony thanked me—which is crazy, 'cause I should be the one thanking them. But he said, "Ruby, thank you for making us all better designers and better people." I could have cried.

I have a new look! For the first time, I am seeing this person come out. I see this girl that I really like, and I'm goin', "Where have you *been*?"

Keepin' the Faith

I pray. I'm a pray-er. I pray every day of my life, and I have people praying for me. And unless you believe, unless you know the power of prayer, you can't go here. There are days where my faith is barely a flicker. I just do not believe I can succeed and I do not feel like anything is working. I am lost. That's the only way I can describe it. It's like I'm walkin' through some strange place and I have no idea where I am supposed to be or how I am supposed to get there. Those are the days when I wish

I could just throw my treadmill out the window. I do not want to lift any weights or even take my bike out for a ride. Literally for thirty minutes, I'm thinking to myself, "What is going to motivate me, because I can't motivate myself?"

So I start praying, and I say, "God, You've got to help me. I can't do this. I can't *do this*." I get all whiny, but God doesn't mind. He knows this is how I get! And then I have a long talk with Him. Sometimes I get mad, saying to Him, "Why did You create me with a body that can stretch the outer limits? What were You thinking?" Other times, I ask Him to please, please, pretty please send me a sign that He knows what I am doing— even if I don't. I just need to know that He sees the bigger picture. He knows why I am the way I am and why I fight so hard, every day of my life. He knows that I do it just to keep on living. We have a good chat; I do most of the talking, but I know He's listening and He will answer my prayers in some way. He will pick me up and give me strength and show me the road. He will get Bertha off the bed and back on the treadmill!

And then the faith kicks in again. Something inside me starts to cheer, "You can do this. You can do this. You *have* to do this. This is your life." And suddenly I feel like I have a purpose again. I do believe that everyone was born for a purpose and a destiny. I feel that no person is insignificant or is a waste or a loser. I feel we all have a job to do. Maybe we don't know what it is, maybe we never quite fulfill that mission a hundred percent, but still, it's there. We're all here for a reason. What's mine? Maybe it's to change the way people think about obesity. Maybe it's to live so I can save other lives. Maybe it's just to be a good friend, daughter, sister, aunt, and to be kind even to strangers who need a nod of acceptance, too, all so that someone else can achieve their purpose as well. God . . . you think You could let me in on your little secret?

This Could Have Been Me

I have just returned from a trip to New York. It was my first time in the city—although it was so quick, I didn't get to see or do anything. I was there to shoot a segment for *Oprah,* and I had no idea flying there that this was going to be so hard! I did not expect to be so moved—and so frightened— by this experience. My heart is still heavy from it. After the first time I was on *Oprah,* her producers called me and asked me to come back on the show. Oprah wanted me to go to the Brookhaven Rehab Center to meet some of the people there. Brookhaven is the last stop for some severely obese people. It really is their last hope. But it can only hold about eighty patients and there are hundreds of people they have to turn down every day. It makes me sick to think that those people will probably die without further help.

I was shocked by what I saw. There were people who were literally so close to death. And all the time I'm thinking, "Ruby, this could have been you." I was in these shoes not so long ago, and it could have been this bad for me. I knew that talking to them might help—both them and me. So I tried my hardest not to think about myself. I tried to focus on the people I was meeting.

I met a man named Dennis there and he was so sweet. I gave him a big hug. He's sixty-one, and he's a husband and a dad of three. His highest weight was 630 pounds. Before going to Brookhaven, he hadn't left his house in a year and he had to depend on his wife for everything, even to take him to the bathroom. This was truly difficult for Dennis because he had always been a hard worker. He had been a banker for thirty-four years! The weight gain and immobility made him depressed, and he finally decided that he had to change; he had to get help. So now he's lost 200 pounds and is still going. He believes he's gonna beat it, and I believe he will, too. He has so much to live for; I told him that.

I also visited with Linda; she's a mom of four kids, and at her biggest, she was 670 pounds. She was also homebound before going to Brookhaven. She was so sad because her kids were getting made fun of at school because of her size. That's what made her come to get help, because she didn't want them to have to suffer because of her. This really hit home for me; I helped raise Georgia's kids, and we're so close, but I didn't want Benjamin or Zachary to be embarrassed. I didn't want kids to say, "Look at your fat aunt." That would have killed me. So I didn't hang around them too much outside. It's not their burden, it's mine to bear.

When I sat down to talk to Oprah, I met this sweet little girl named Marina, whose mama, Renee, weighed nearly 900 pounds. She couldn't even get out of bed. Well, Marina said to us, "I didn't even see my mother that way. I didn't see her as that big. I just loved her. She was my best friend." Renee decided to get gastric bypass surgery and it took eight men from the fire department just to get her out of her home. Twelve days after the surgery, her heart gave out and she passed on. Well, this broke my heart. Not just that Renee died and left behind these two beautiful girls, but that the people who loved her didn't just see the shell. They really saw the person inside. My friends are always telling me, "Ruby, you are so beautiful. You are so sexy." Even when I was 700 pounds! Are they trying to make me feel good—or is that what they really see? Well, after meeting Marina, I know that it's possible that's what they see; if you love someone, you can see through to their soul. That's the power of love. I wish that more people could do this. I wish more people could see what I see when I look at those people in Brookhaven. I see mothers and fathers and wives and husbands and sisters and brothers. I see good, gentle, caring, courageous people that deserve to be happy and healthy and *living*. I don't see freaks. I see a lot of Rubys—wanting so badly to change, not knowing how, but dreaming of that day and praying it becomes a reality.

Living My Best Life: A Letter to Oprah Winfrey

Dear Oprah:
Where do I begin to thank you? You already know that you are my idol. Not only have you personally inspired me for so long,

but then you went and asked me to be on your show, not once, but twice! For years you have worked to make the world a better place. And you really have. Day in and day out you move people to improve the quality of their lives: to feel better, to live longer, and to be healthier in mind, body, and spirit. You have taught so many of us to strive for what we dream about. It has been my heart's cry that people be saved from this addiction I am fighting and you gave me an unbelievable opportunity to bring awareness of it on your show. You really understand what I am going through on a personal level, as you have battled weight very publicly yourself. I know you are wanting to lose weight again these days, and if that is important to your health and well-being, then I know you will. I just wanted to repeat what you've taught us all many times: we are not defined by our size or a number on a scale. We are defined by what lives inside. And there isn't anyone on this planet who doesn't know Oprah is beautiful any way you look at her! I sat next to you and I was thinking, "She glows, y'all! She really glows." The beauty of changing lives—saving lives—like you do every day, far outweighs anything a scale could ever say.

So thank you again for all that you do for people and for all that you did for me—especially for sending me to Brookhaven. It opened my eyes!

With gratitude,
Ruby Gettinger

Now I'm Cookin'!

So here's my deal with Dr. Bradley. He said that if I dropped below the 350-pound mark, we would start to ease back on my Ourlife prepackaged meals. Well, I am there, and I am holding him to his word! These meals have been great for me, but I also need to know that I can take care of myself. I am now changing to the five-day plan, where I eat their meals for lunch and dinner, Monday through Friday. I am on my own for breakfast every day (just oatmeal for now) and totally off on weekends. This is a big responsibility for me, but I am up for it. I am cooking for myself! Jeff is fallin' down laughing at this moment because he cannot remember the last time I turned my stove on. He says, "You sure you know how to work it? You're not gonna burn down the house, are you?" Well, I'll show him!

I am so excited! There is no one telling me what to eat, so I have to make the right choices. But the good thing is that I feel like I have learned so much about nutrition now, I can do it. I can read labels, I can cook without oil and butter. I just have to remember that "fried" is not a basic food group! Dr. Bradley is giving me some great recipes I can make. Here are two I am trying this weekend (cross fingers, y'all!):

GRILLED BALSAMIC CHICKEN SALAD

Serves 4 (so, Jeff and Jim and Georgia . . . you are eatin'
this with me!)

1 pound romaine lettuce leaves, torn
1¼ pounds chicken breast halves without skin

Marinade in 1¾ cups balsamic dressing (see ingredients below) for 2 hours, grill 2 minutes on both sides till done, cool, and slice over greens.

Balsamic Marinade

¾ cup water
¼ cup balsamic vinegar
⅛ cup lime juice
1 tsp Dijon mustard
1 tsp capers
1 tsp Italian seasoning
1 tsp garlic
1 fluid ounce olive oil
salt and pepper, as needed

Dressing for Salad

1/16 cup balsamic vinegar
⅛ cup vegetable oil
½ tbsp garlic, chopped

½ tbsp Italian seasoning

salt and pepper, as needed

TOPPINGS FOR SALAD

¼ cup walnuts, toasted

1 cup grape tomatoes

¼ cup Craisins

4 ounces reduced-fat cheddar cheese, white, sharp, small dice

CHESAPEAKE CRAB CAKES

Serves 4

¾ pound crabmeat, back fin

½ pound crabmeat, special

1 tbsp garlic, chopped

½ tbsp Old Bay seafood seasoning

¼ cup Egg Beaters 99 percent egg substitute, pasteurized

½ cup light mayonnaise

1½ tbsp Dijon mustard

½ tsp Tabasco sauce

1 tbsp Worcestershire sauce

⅛ cup white wine

½ tsp paprika

½ cup panko (Japanese bread crumbs)

salt and pepper, as needed

Mix all ingredients below in mixing bowl, then gently fold in crabmeat, forming 3-ounce cakes. Bake at 425 degrees for 10 to 12 minutes.

I remember all the wonderful times we had growing up together. Ruby was the brightest light that shone all around us. She never let one ugly word tarnish her spirit and determination to be an example for others to follow. We were together every day for many years. We used to go to the playground and the boys would roll us around in big truck tires and we would scream to the top of our lungs until the tire toppled over and came to a rest. We would swing on the swings and laugh and play. She was such a tomboy! We had the same little pixie haircut for several years. Then, as we grew and got older and became teenagers, her weight became a real issue, but she still kept that same glowing personality. She used to say, "Just look at my beautiful face" and she'd laugh! Ruby, your face IS beautiful and so is your soul— through all of the good and bad, you persevere and never let anything get you down.

I remember one time when we were in church: Ruby sat down on the pew with us and it cracked. She crawled out on the floor of the church so she wouldn't get in trouble (it didn't work!). It pained me that sometimes people were so cruel to her: like at that restaurant when our waitress was so rude about the weight. Well, we had to tell that waitress off. We made her so mad that she called the police on us. We ran outside and made faces at her through the window.

Although Ruby laughs all the time, and pretends it doesn't bother her, I know that sometimes her heart was heavy. Ruby told us once that she thought she was gonna die before she turned thirty, but that God wouldn't let it happen until she got to tell her story to the world. Well, Ruby . . . thirty has passed, and you are now getting to tell your AMAZING story to the world. You deserve the best that life has to offer because you are such a giving person, generous to everyone that you meet.

—*Julie*

RUBY'S DIARY

12   LET'S GET PHYSICAL

The Start of Something New

I am in a rut. I am so unmotivated these days to work out; I'm bored! I know Reese is amazing, and he knows his stuff, but all he has me do is the treadmill and the weights and it's killing my knees. I am finding it harder and harder to get through my workouts. I know he wants me to up the intensity, but the whole time, I am zoning out. I just don't care. I want to bicycle so bad, but Reese keeps saying, "Stick to the plan." Well, I'm tired of sticking. I feel stuck. Now I want to try something new.

Dr. Bradley had a suggestion. He set this meeting up for me with this New York "guru," Edward Jackowski. He wrote a book called *Escape Your Shape*. So this doctor, he holds nothing back; he tells it like he sees it (must be a New York thing). He said to me, "You wanna lose weight, then you are going about it all wrong." He told me it's not that I need to be upping the intensity like Reese says, I need to be changing my workout. He says I am an hourglass, and because of my shape, I don't need to lift weights. Sounds good to me! He put me on a recumbent bike and I loved it. I was going so fast—and my knees didn't hurt. He made me really rethink my whole routine.

So the next day I woke up and I was hurting so bad I could not move. I had to call Jeff to help me get out of my bed. This new workout made me realize I had muscles in places I didn't know existed—and every one of them was screaming. I knew I had to talk to Reese and his partner, Erin. I had to tell them that I wanted to try different things. So we sat down, and I could see by the look in their faces they were not liking one word of it. I felt terrible. I hate conflict and hurting people's feelings. Reese has helped me so much, and I owe him a lot. But I can't go lower on my calories, so it's my workout that has to change. I gotta go crazy on it to lose more weight and lose it faster. I said I wanted to try Pilates and Erin was like, "I don't see you doing that." But I couldn't understand. Why doesn't she see me doing it? If not that, why can't I ride a bike or box—or dance for that matter? Why can't I go out there and be creative? There's a whole world out there. There's nothing that says I have to only work out in a gym. I love being outdoors; I love the sun on my face, the wind in my hair, and the sound of the birds and the ocean in my ears. I am seeing no sun at all in this gym! I feel like I'm not just on a machine, I *am* a machine!

Well, I don't know if they got what I was saying. But if they didn't hear me, that's okay, too; I have to hear myself. Both of us made a stand. Reese said he was only going to train me if it was his way. Well, I respect that. I really do. His commitment and passion is one of the things I really like about him. But even though I understood, I thought it was best if we parted ways. In the end, I had to say good-bye to them. It was so hard to do! We hugged and Reese said, "I hope you come back." But as I walked out, I realized that I wasn't walking away from him so much as I was walking toward the opportunity to make my own choices. I needed to be out on my own now. It's totally up to me to find new exercises that are gonna motivate me to stay on course. I'm gonna show them. And not just them. I'm gonna show myself. I know I'm right about this, because in the past, when I lost the motivation, that's when I gave up. But I'm also afraid. Change is scary. When things are going so well, why rock the boat?

And Reese really did help make things go well for a long time.

I guess part of how I'm growing is that I'm learning more about myself and what I need and want. The trick is not to get bored. I need to be outside. I need to be doing cardio. I need something I enjoy and love. It has to be fun. I want to try every kind of exercise I can until I find something that makes me excited to work out three or four times a week. So bring it on!

Row, Row, Row Your Boat

Three of my really good friends—Danna, Chris, and Toni—were in town to spend a girls' weekend with Georgia and me. I was so excited to see them all! I've known them since we were teenagers together. Even though we're older now and life has pulled us in different directions, we're all still really close. We try to get together at least once a year to catch up, hang out, talk about the hubbies and the kids. The three married ones always need an update from me and Georgia on the trials of being single in our thirties so we give them an earful.

The last time my girls saw me, I was well over five hundred pounds. Whenever they used to come for a reunion, everything revolved around food, so I was nervous at first. We used to go out to eat, then after that, we'd head to the grocery store to stock up on snacks. We'd just sit around all weekend laughing, giggling, telling stories, and (you guessed it) stuffing our faces.

But this time, I was determined not to fall back into old habits. I wanted to show them all the new Ruby! There would be food—but it was going to be *healthy*. And instead of just sitting around, shooting the breeze, we were gonna get out and have some fun. I had it all worked out.

I sent Georgia to pick them up from the airport as usual. When they got out of the car, you should have seen their faces. I lost over 250 pounds since they last saw me, and they could not believe their eyes. They just stood there dumbfounded. It didn't take long before we all started crying like babies. It confirmed that my journey was real: my friends were seeing the change in me. I was proud, but I needed to get the weekend rolling if we were gonna do everything I wanted to. Enough tears, ladies, it's time to laugh!

We left Savannah with me behind the wheel of Jeff's Jeep. It was wild! I used to always make somebody else drive, and insist that the air conditioner be on full blast. But this time I was driving from Savannah to Tybee Island—and in a five-speed stick shift! The doors were off, the top was down, I popped the clutch and off we went. I never heard us laugh or scream as hard as we did when I ripped out of the driveway.

I have been friends with these four amazing women more than half my life, and we have spent many weekends together, but as we were heading down the highway with the wind blowing through our hair, I realized that this was the first time I was truly able to be physically and completely a part of what was going on. Until that moment, I had always been on the sidelines, cheering my beautiful friends on, giving them advice, sharing their joys and heartaches . . . but now I was experiencing the same things as they were. Somehow I knew this was going to be a life-altering weekend.

The girls were all shocked when I was the first one out of bed in the morning and eating a healthy breakfast. They were in for an even bigger surprise when we headed to the beach for a workout with my trainer, Shazia. We spent a full hour dancing in the sand, throwing a medicine ball around, and doing aerobics. There is nothing like working out on the beach! When we were good and tired, everybody wanted to take a nap before heading to the salon for a pedicure and manicure. But I said, "No way, ladies . . . we are going kayaking!" You should have seen their jaws drop. They looked at me as if I had lost my mind.

I have to admit, I didn't give a whole lot of thought to how packed the day was gonna be when I was doing the scheduling. I just knew I wanted to take a chance and try something different. I called around, found a rental place with instructors that ensured me they had kayaks a 350-pound woman could fit into. They also said they'd send someone to teach me what to do. I was really looking forward to this . . . until I saw that itty-bitty yellow plastic boat. How was I gonna fit into that? I wanted to cry. All the memories of being too fat to do anything came flooding back. I worried about what would happen if I tipped the kayak over. I thought about a lifetime of being too heavy for the rides at the amusement park, about breaking every beach chair I had ever sat on, and about the constant search to find a seat my size—any seat! I was frozen for a few minutes. But then I decided that my girlfriends had come all this way to see the new me. I wasn't gonna stand there humidified. So I took a deep breath and tried to relax (yeah, right!). I listened to the instructors. Then my friends took my hands and helped me lean back in the water. The next thing I know, I'm wedged in that tiny boat and it's not so bad. It was actually comfy. Who woulda thought?

This was a milestone for me! After decades of being an

observer, I was about to be a participant. I was in the game! Those uggy days are behind me now. For the first time ever, I was fully living life, not just seeing it race by.

I quickly learned how to paddle. We all I rowed around and around, racing and laughing and loving every minute of it. No one told me how hard paddling would be or what it would make my muscles feel like, but I didn't mind the pain. It reminded me that I was alive!

After we had enough, we headed back to the beach. We must have been a sight—all of us hugging and crying. I was so proud that my friends were there to share this day with me. I know in my heart that if they hadn't been by my side supporting me, I never would have had the strength to try any of it.

Before we left, there was one more thing I knew I had to do while I had the courage. My entire life, I've been terrified of the sea. I never liked dipping so much as my big toe into it. Kayaking today seemed safer to me than standing in the ocean, even just up to my ankles. But I knew that if I had just paddled around in the deep water for hours, then there was no reason why I couldn't stand for a minute and feel the waves lap against me and envelop me just once.

I asked the girls if they would come out with me, but they insisted that this was something I had to do on my own. I slowly stepped out into the cold Atlantic ocean, baby step by baby step. I waded out until the water was barely above my knees. It was freezing. I knew there was just one thing to do—so I took a deep breath and lunged forward. I went under and held my breath for a few seconds before finally coming back up to the surface. When I did, I realized that I was floating. Because I still weighed over three hundred pounds, my body was buoyant. I just laid back and let myself go. I lay there with my eyes closed. I could feel the sun shining down, too. I was calmer than I had ever been before.

There I was, floating in the ocean. A far cry from 716 pounds. Although I still had a couple hundred pounds left to go before reaching my goal weight, I was happy. I was enjoying true freedom! It was the most wonderful and amazing experience I had ever had. The girls were all standing on the shore crying. I know I was, too.

Having a Ball

I played tennis today! I never thought I would be able to run around a court, chasing after such an itty-bitty ball, but I did it. And I couldn't believe how good I was the first time! I played with Amy Bradley, who is a major pro. She thinks I am very athletic and a natural. She wants me to get on a team. WHO? Is she crazy? Well, I could not wait for us to take on Brittany and Georgia, because I wanted to kick their butts! I never realized it, but I do have a little competitive streak in me. I don't like to admit that, because it makes me feel mean and petty, but I guess it's true because I did *not* want to let them win! Every time those two would score a point against me, they would do this little happy dance. And it just made my blood boil! I warned them. I said, "If you do the dance, y'all are gonna go down!" I was so focused. I was so determined. There was no ball that was getting past me. They were going down, down, down! And that's what happened. They won one, and we won the rest. We were the champions. I loved beating them. Is that terrible to say? I just can't help it, because this feeling is an incredible high. I loved being a winner. If I feel this great killing my girlfriends on the tennis court, can you imagine how good I will feel when I kick the butt of my food addiction? This was a *good* day! I want play again tomorrow. I want to challenge everyone. I know I'm getting cocky, but it feels so good . . . and I think my friends will forgive me because they're a little competitive sometimes, too.

I Like to Move It, Move It . . .

So I am loving my exercising these days! I don't even mind that there is a lot of it, or that sometimes it is hard, hard, hard. I almost can't believe it. It's all because Drew and Shazia make it fun and they switch it up from day to day. When I met them, it was love at first workout. The best part is the "tag-team training." I get to spend time with both of them—they have such different personalities—and I get the benefit of what each knows best. They are the funnest people you will ever meet. And I love that their studio is designed to accommodate all sizes. It is "Rubyfied"! I can use the equipment and not worry about my weight breaking it like I do in some other gyms. And all of the chairs are armless, so I can always be comfy when I sit. It's like from the moment I met these two, they got me. I think I'm blabbering on and on. It's just that I saw so many other trainers and they were all incredible and each taught me something, but I'm just so excited about Drew and Shazia that I chose them. I felt this instant connection with them. They like to have a good time like me, but they can be serious when they have to be. They also *listen* to what I am saying and feeling. They're gonna push me, but they're gonna push me in a direction that makes sense for *me*.

For now, they are asking me to get in at least thirty minutes of cardio per day. My goal is to be able to do forty-five minutes at some point in the future. I am supposed to do this for a minimum of four days a week, until I can handle doing it six days a week. That is a lot of cardio! Then I also strength-train at least two days a week. My aim is to work up to doing that four days a week.

I am supposed to do at least one activity each day. The idea is just to keep moving. What I love is that this can mean dancing, walking, biking, lifting, swimming, or any other activity that gets my heart rate up. They also tell me that it keeps my body in a "metabolic state," which means I am constantly burning calories and fat. (I can't believe all the science I am learning!) It all sounds good to me, but the most important part is that I love exercise now. I wake up in the morning and I want to work out! That is a major change for me. I do not even feel like being lazy. I am having fun, and I am not bored anymore. I feel like I have so many options.

• • •

Of course, I would like to see the numbers on the scale go down quicker. I'm just impatient. I want to get to my goal weight quick. My mind is set. But my team tells me that my weight loss will depend on a lot of things, including how often I work out, how long, and how hard—and how much I stick with my meal plan. It's also real important that I drink four thirty-two-ounce containers of water each day. I am sweatin' a lot! Drew and Shazia tell me that there will be weeks where I will lose nothing (I could cry . . .), and then there may be some weeks where I lose more than expected (woo-hoo!), but they have given me a general range to shoot for each week. I've also been warned that the smaller I get, the harder it will be to keep the pounds coming off. I live in fear of a plateau, but I know when I hit it, my team will hit it back hard. We'll find a way to get over the hump.

Basically, my workout changes every session. I never know what's in store, and that is exciting. Sometimes they toss me a big ol' medicine ball (like playing catch); other times we're biking, boxing, or doing cheerleading moves (Go Ruby! Go Ruby!). Drew and Shazia asked me to keep a cardio log so I can see my progress and make sure I am getting in enough of the right types of exercises. When I look at this log, I see that I really am stretching myself slowly but surely. One of the first times I exercised, I wrote, "I did 20 sit-ups today." That was more than a month ago. Yesterday's entry was way better than that! I'm up to 108 sit-ups! I am very impressed with myself. The plan they worked out may not be right for everyone, but it is just right for me. So here is what they had me do today. I get tuckered out just writing about it, but I want to keep all this in my head 'cause the goal is to one day be able to walk into a gym anywhere and do my own thing. This all is a good model for me on that day!

My Current Workout

1. Warm up with 10 minutes of boxing
2. Resistance Training:
   - Lat Pulldowns: 10–20 reps / 40–70 pounds / 2–3 sets
   - Seated Rows: 10–20 reps / 40–70 pounds / 2–3 sets
   - Inclined Chest Press on Smith Machine: 10–20 reps / 30–50 pounds / 2–3 sets
   - Shoulder Press: 10–20 reps / 8–15 pounds / 2–3 sets
   - Dumbbell or Resistance-Band Biceps Curls: 10–20 reps / 8–15 pounds / 2–3 sets
   - Rope Pulldowns or Overhead Dumbell Extensions: 10–20 reps / 8–20 pounds / 2–3 sets
   - Leg Extensions with Ankle Weights: 20–30 reps / 5–10 pounds / 2–3 sets
   - Seated Leg Curls with Band Behind Ankle: 20–30 reps / 5–15 pounds / 2–3 sets

3. Dance Routine (20–30 minutes). This is so much fun, it's not even like a real workout. I feel like I am in a club, partying!

4. Abs: My favorite, the Crunch and Punch! Because I can't get down on the floor (I would never be able to get up), my trainers came up with an abs routine for me that involves sitting on a bench, with or without incline. I do crunches and sit-ups while punching at their boxing mitts.

I wonder what Drew and Shazia first thought when I came huffing and puffing into their studio. They were probably thinking, "Lord, what are we getting ourselves into?!" But they are good people, and I love that they "get me." They sense when motivation is slipping and they are constantly coming up with fun new ways to get me excited and on my feet. They have changed the way I think about exercise. It's not a chore for me anymore; it's something that makes me feel good. It's empowering! I asked them to talk about that first day I knocked on their door . . . and where they see me going . . .

A Note from Ruby's Trainers

When Ruby first arrived at the fitness studio for the audition training session, we didn't know what to expect. The first thing that made a strong impression was her climb up the stairs to meet us. It took her almost twenty minutes to get up one flight of steps! We knew immediately that her knees and stamina were going to be limiting factors in training her. When she came through that door, however, all of the limitations went out the window. Her personality and positive energy filled the room! We immediately connected with her. As trainers, we know that you have to have the desire and determination to overcome your limitations in order to reach your goals. Ruby has those two qualities! Her knees and stamina have never stopped her from moving forward in life and in every workout we have had with her. I mean, come on, that girl can really move!

In our short time with her, she has crossed many milestones. She can now fly up a flight of stairs! She has walked over three miles without stopping! She has completed 180 crunches in one workout! She lost thirty-two pounds in a month and a half! Those are not ordinary results, but it can happen. The great thing is that she actually looks forward to exercising! And we look forward to training her! We're a match made in heaven.

Our goal for Ruby is to get her to a point where she can maintain a healthy lifestyle on her own. We want her to be healthy, happy, and comfortable in her own skin. We want her to be capable of walking into a fitness center with all of the knowledge necessary to work out on her own. We want her to be able to enjoy all of the activities life has to offer! No limitations!

We want the best for you, Ruby,
Drew and Shazia Edmonds

13 CHILDHOOD HOPES AND DREAMS

The Two Faces of Ruby Gettinger

I have hundreds of pounds to lose, but today it feels like I have thousands. My friends say there are two types of Ruby: Normal Ruby and Diet Ruby. Today I am Diet Ruby. I am grumpy. I am buggin'. I am frustrated. If anybody says anything to annoy me or just looks at me funny, I am gonna bite their head off. (How many calories do you think an adult-size head has?!) Really, that's how irritable I feel. Why? Because it's taking so much work for me to get healthy, and I need to feel and see a difference, but I don't. I look in the mirror and I don't see any of it. I look at every angle, and it all looks the same: *big!* When I work out it hurts, and it's not getting any easier. Everything about this diet is driving me nuts lately. And this is not just about me; it's not like I can just say, "The helicopter with it" because a lot of people have put a lot of time and effort into helping me and a lot of people are watching me, trying to change their lives, too. I want to beat this thing so I can look at people suffering from the same kind of Beast as I am and tell them they can do it, too! They really can. I can't say that to them right now because I haven't reached my goal yet. But I feel like everybody is telling me what to do, and it's making me mad. I'm so sick of it! I gotta change what I eat, how much I eat, and when I eat. I knew it would be hard, but this is really getting me down; it's knocking me to the ground. I am scared that I won't be able to keep it up. I am scared that I am setting myself up to fail again. Honest to God, I really feel like this is my last chance. I can't let it go.

A Dark and Stormy Night

The sky really matched my mood today. It was dark and stormy and angry. So I went out on the porch to watch what it would do. It's strange, but I love storms. I always have. I was feeling a little happier when I saw the lightning strike like fireworks, but then a tornado siren sounded and we lost all the power in the house. I was with Jim and Ben, and we had to get inside fast. The safest place you can go in a tornado is the bathtub. But I can't fit there. If I got down, I wouldn't be able to get up. So the kids and the dogs were in the tub, and I was out in the hallway by myself. I was trying to put on a brave face for them, calling out and saying, "It's okay." But my heart was beating so fast. I was scared. I was panicked. I felt so helpless. For the first time, I realized that if a tornado came, I couldn't hide anywhere. I would die. I never thought about it before—not until I saw the boys' faces. Jim said, "Ruby you have to lose weight because I can't lose you." Until now I never saw how my situation could cause others so much fear. I'm hurting myself, but I'm also hurting the people closest to me. I am in a freakin' cage. Just what I needed, one more thing for me to be afraid of: tornadoes.

Fear is such a big part of my life. I am afraid of remembering my past. I am afraid of getting hurt if I work out too hard. I am terrified of the unknown. Dr. Brewerton says I am a pain avoider. Well, who isn't?! But there is something in my past that I fear. Something that is just too painful for me to remember. What in the helicopter is it? Did it sabotage my weight? My whole life? Did it scare the crapiola out of me so bad that I had to block it out? There's something there, I know it. There's something I am deathly afraid of. Or is it just the unknown I'm afraid of? When am I going to deal with this?

Picture This

I went to my sister Jamie's house today. I am so blessed to have her and Steve—the best brother-in-law ever—as family. They are both beautiful, beautiful people. And their daughter, Karen, my niece, my heart, is so beautiful and amazing, too. Jamie is doing what she can to help me. She even took out a bunch of pictures to try to jog my memory about my childhood. We were sitting in her kitchen, going through my past, and she was telling me stories, lots of stories, about me and my siblings growing up. NOTHING was coming back to me. It was like she was talking about a complete stranger. I do not remember any of the things that she said I used to do. I do not remember going to any of the places she said we used to play. Not even one of them. She told me that I would try to please my daddy so hard even though I was already his little girl. I would climb up the monkey bars to try and show off for him. She said I would have blisters on my hands from doing it over and over so much. I looked at the photos and all I thought is, "Who is this angry little girl?" I look so mad in every picture. Jamie is in all these cute, pretty little dresses, smiling, but I look like a boy. All I remember is this general sense of loving my life. So if I was so happy, how did I get to be 700 pounds? Part of me really wants to remember these stories Jamie is telling me, and part of me is scared to death that if I do, it might trigger some other memories, some bad or traumatic ones. So maybe I am better off not knowing? Maybe if I unleashed those memories, it would be even worse than *not* knowing? But I gotta know. I gotta shine a light in all my dark places if I am ever going to beat this.

The Music Man

I had a breakthrough today: I remembered something from childhood, something really vivid that I never recalled before. I don't know what triggered it or how it happened, but it was thrilling. I was sitting at the hospital with my daddy, looking at him and praying for him to get better when suddenly I saw the hand of a child playing a violin. I flashed back to what I thought was a music teacher—a man who looked like he could be German or from somewhere like Germany, and he had a beard. I knew I knew him from somewhere. Georgia came in to see daddy, so I told her about it. She was real excited for me . . . until I told her the rest of my memory. I said, "I think his name was Rumpelstiltskin!" "Ruby," she said, "are you kidding me? Are you pulling my leg? There is no Rumpelstiltskin except in a fairy tale!" She was mad because she thought that I was joking her, but I was deathly serious. I had to prove to her—and myself—that I am not crazy. I told her to call all the music schools around because I know this is a real memory, not something my head is making up. I called my mother, but she had no memory of me ever playing the violin either. Then I spoke to Jamie, who said, "Yes! I remember your violin recitals—they were really boring." Jamie, Mom, and Georgia had a big laugh at the name Rumpelstiltskin. Then Jamie went home and told my brother-in-law Steve, who recalled that there was a music teacher named Mr. Rumple. He said that he was a German man and that we kids used to tease him and call him Rumpelstiltskin. Steve remembered it plain as day.

I am not sure what this memory means, if anything at all, but I am convinced it's the start of me breaking down my walls. If I can see one thing in the past, I know the rest will come into focus, too. I am so excited, but I am also scared. Every day, I never know what I might remember—whether it'll be a good thing or a bad thing. But the fact that something, anything, is coming back to me . . . that gives me hope.

Uggy People

Georgia and I used to hit the roads and stay out most of the night with our girlfriends. Even though most people assumed we were party animals, we were having good, clean fun. We were talking today about how we used to drive to these gay bars when we were teenagers. And the way we found them was because Danna, Georgia, and I would see the cutest guy and we'd want to meet him and hang out. The next thing we knew, all our crushes were gay! So let me tell you, some of the sexiest guys are gay! Even though I couldn't date them, we became the best of friends! We couldn't go in these places because we were too young, but we loved talking with the drag queens out in the parking lot. We got to know them; they were our friends; we loved them! We loved their style. We knew every one of them on a first-name basis. Well, one night, we were out late, driving around near one of these clubs, and this cop pulled us over. He had been following us for a few days and we had no idea. He said to me, "I've been watching you. I see all these people coming in and out of your home all times of day and night. You have these beautiful girls and guys coming and going; why would they hang out with *you*?" I didn't know what he meant. I was so scared he was gonna arrest me, I wasn't even hearing what he said. Georgia started to talk back, to defend me. She said, "We hang out with her because we have a good time." But the cop was mean. He said, "You're lying." Then he turned to me and accused me of being a drug dealer! ME! Like that is the only reason ANYONE would want to be around someone as hideous as me. He went through my car, my trunk; he searched everything. Well, we were scared to death. And he kept saying, "No big, heavy girl like you is gonna have thin, pretty friends who want to hang out with you—you're doing something for them. You're giving them something . . ." He kept it going for an hour. Then I think, because he couldn't find anything suspicious, he gave up. We were shaking. I could not get over it. Georgia, Danna, Chris, and I were so frightened! Here was this police officer— he was supposed to be a good, moral person who protects people. And every other one I ever met is. But he wasn't. He was harassing me, accusing me, and insulting me like I was a piece of trash. I will never forget it. It made Georgia cry when I brought it up today, although it's gotta be more than twenty years ago now. Some things just stay with you.

Baby Talk

I saw a baby in a stroller out in the park today and she was so cute. She couldn't have been more than six months old. Part of me believes that anything is possible; I am all about proving that. But I can't ever let myself think that I can have a child. If I do, I am just hurting myself. My friends see me with kids and they ask, "Ruby, are you getting the itch?" It hurts, because I will always have "the itch." There was a time in my life when having a baby was on my wish list. At the very top. I love babies; I wanted to have four or five of them. Maybe even six! But I think I just don't have that option anymore. My addiction shut the door on that dream. My doctor told me that getting pregnant at this current weight could be life-theatening. I'm in love with children. I love all my friends' kids and I am the best aunt you will ever find (partly because I have the best niece and nephew you will ever find!). God blessed me when He surrounded me with so many sweet, innocent, loving children. Hanging out with my angels Karen, Jim, Zach, Maryanna, and Gracie the other day was great! We always have a good time when we're together. Sometimes I think that I would love to open a huge orphanage. I could be with children and babies all day long, and I could hold them and play with them and take care of them. I think this is a great idea, but Jeff has to be the voice of reason, again. He always says, "What if someone wants to adopt them? Isn't that what an orphanage does? How could you let them go?" And I know he's right; I couldn't handle it. I couldn't give my heart out like that to those kids and then just lose them. So for now, my Foxy and Lucy are my babies; they're my children. They were a gift from Georgia, Ben, and Zach. They came from the same parents but were born a year apart. One has been with me for ten years, and the other one nine. We are together night and day. They are so smart, they understand everything I'm saying. Foxy is the queen of the house. She acts like she was born with a golden spoon! And Lucy is a child at heart, a little rebel who loves to play, play, play! I can't imagine or even fathom ever being without them. I pray God will let them live as long as I do! The joy they give me is just so great.

Speaking of little ones, my friend Melissa and her husband, Michael, recently had a baby, so we all went to L.A. to throw them a little shower. Traveling for me is always very stressful. I am a big girl in a little world, so flying is hard for me. I have to make sure someone I know is booked next to me. So Jim volunteered to be squished this time. But this trip was worse than most: they told me that as a safety precaution, I had to have two seats. The whole front of the plane heard it! I had to move to another row and they made Jim go to the back of the plane. Everybody was looking. I was humidified. I was up front and all my friends were way behind me. I was miserable *and* lonely.

When we got to L.A., we met our friends Tomas and Irina and we went to Knott's Berry Farm Amusement Park. I used to take them there all the time when they were kids. Well, it's just not the place for me now. I can't fit on most of the rides, there is food everywhere, and I can't walk around all day 'cause I get worn out. Plus, there are these great funnel cakes! Deep-fried funnel cakes are the best, especially with whipped cream. I could have cried 'cause they smelled so good! That was one of the highlights of my trip. WHO ADMITS THAT? I am scared for me. LOL!

While everyone was having fun on the roller coaster, I was just watching them, wondering what would it feel like to go upside down and do all those fast twists and turns? I saw them all screaming and laughing; I can't wait for the day when I can go with them. When will I be able to do that? Will I *ever* be able to do that? I know it's just a silly ride, but it was just one more thing I couldn't do. One more limitation for Ruby.

I was having a terrible time walking around; I just got exhausted and my knees were killing me. So we rented a moped chair for me to drive around the park in. Well, when I sat in it, it broke. I bent the thingy that holds the wheel; it just gave under my weight. No rides, no mopeds, there wasn't anything that I could ride on! My friends seemed to think that I could do the log ride. They thought it would hold me, and frankly, I was willing to give it a try, because I was getting so down. The log *looked* sturdy and the seats seemed roomy enough for me to squeeze Bertha into, so I tried. But when it started to move, I panicked. I was scared to death thinking that all this weight was gonna tilt us over and break our necks—or worse, drown us! I thought we would flip over for sure. But thank God, I didn't flip the log, and I had fun after all. I felt like a normal person for just a few minutes that day. It was a good memory to take home after all.

Anyway, I'm happy for my friends because they have such a sweet little baby. That baby's lips are beautiful. I swear I am in love. I just wanted to take him home with me. I was holding him, and I could see Georgia looking at me like she could read my mind. She thinks I want a baby of my own. I don't know what skinny Ruby's gonna want when I get to that point. But sometimes I ask myself, "Could I actually be a mother one day?" I've always been like a mother to Foxy and Lucy, Karen, Ben, Zach, Jim, Gary, Miles, Matthew, Gracie, Graham, Maryanna and Manly, Anna, Katcha, Irina, Tomas, Ryland, and so many others. Every step closer I get to losing the weight, the more possibilities open up for me. I might ride a roller coaster. I might do a lot of things I never thought I'd be able to do before. So for now I find comfort in thinking, maybe, just maybe . . .

In Memory of Lucy

Sadly, just as this book was going to press, my beloved Lucy passed away. Lucy was my youngest "child," my heart. Our time was taken too soon. She had the sweetest eyes I have ever seen; she was, as I have said many times, my rebel. Foxy and I will miss her every second of the day. A piece of my heart has left with her.

I met Ruby almost twenty years ago (I hope that doesn't give away her age, because she would KILL me if I told anyone that!). I had just moved to Savannah and was working at the mall. She came into my store, and we connected immediately. We must have talked for an hour, laughing and getting to know each other, right there in the middle of The Gap, while I was supposed to be folding shirts or ringing up purchases or something (Ruby does have a knack for getting you into mischief!). I found out later that she was really on a secret mission for a friend of hers named Greg. Greg had seen me in the store and wanted to meet me, but he valued Ruby's opinion so much that he wanted to know what she thought of me before he introduced himself. So she walked into that store and proceeded to basically interview me, and I didn't even know it! All I knew was this very large girl with the most beautiful smile had me laughing my head off and soon I was sharing my secrets with her. We've been the best of friends ever since, and I'm sure many people who know Ruby would have a similar story. Maybe not the spying part, although she is a pretty good matchmaker (Greg and I have been married for seventeen years thanks to her), but the part where you feel you could tell her anything and everything. In fact, I believe it's because of God's plan for her: people open up to her because she's really here to help others.

When I met Ruby, she immediately questioned me about whether I went to church. As our friendship grew, she would talk to me about my relationship with God and take me to her church.

I had never seen someone so sure of their faith. It brings tears to my eyes to think about it. Not only did she introduce me to my wonderful husband, Greg, but she introduced me to my faith. Literally, our friendship completely changed my life. That is what is so amazing about Ruby. She encouraged me and loved me and helped me become a better person. I laugh thinking about the times she has given me advice on my marriage or on parenting my seven children! Here she is, a single woman with two Yorkies for children, and she is giving ME practical advice on how to be a better wife and mom. The strange thing is, it's always great advice!

But I know that her life has not always been all laughs. This world would like to steal away her joy; she and her family have endured so much over the years, and yet she still clings to hope. Even with the trials in her life, she has always been a dreamer at heart. She has dreamed of helping others who struggle with addictions, wanting to help those who most people would consider hopeless. Instead of being consumed with self-pity for her situations, she fiercely defends her friends and does everything she can to provide the best for those she loves. She never takes people for granted and is so thankful when someone does even the tiniest thing for her. I guess that's what sets her apart from other people: she can see past someone's faults and see their potential, then she encourages them to be that better person. Imagine if everyone was like that: nonjudgmental and compassionate. That's what Ruby is about; she is a treasure.

—Leslie

14   ALMOST FAMOUS

R-E-S-P-E-C-T

I was in Myrtle Beach today with Denny, just walking on the boardwalk, and we could hardly take one step without people stopping me, wanting to tell me all about their own struggles—and many of these struggles weren't even weight-related. A lot were about the different kinds of addictions there are—and there are many! I got stopped by kids, too—some as young as five and six years old. They were waving and calling out to me! We share so many of the same concerns. They are just looking to make changes in their lives and I can relate in ways lots of other people can't. I'm easy to spot on the street these days. I'm pretty hard to miss. It must be the red hair, don't you think? LOL. At first, I thought just local people in Savannah would stop me. But nuh-uh, it is everywhere. It doesn't matter where we go these days. People even stop Georgia, Denny, Jeff, and especially Jim to talk about how to be a better friend to people struggling with our issues. (Though when Georgia got a makeover with a new hair color, she kind of threw some people off!) The amazing thing about getting stopped is how many of the people who talk to me simply want me to call a friend or family member on the phone to give them some words of inspiration, comfort, or advice. We really are all in this together. One woman asked me to call her sister because she is so big, and she has tried every diet and it doesn't work. Now she's got diabetes. Every time it's the same: they dial and hand me the phone and I go, "Hey!" The person on the other end instantly knows who it is. They know my voice and they are now getting to know my message. I really just want people to pay attention to what I'm saying. I want them to listen. So I don't mind them coming up to me everywhere I go. I don't mind any of it, because it means people respect me. I really want to create respect for *all* the Rubys out there.

There was one moment, though, this past Christmas, when doing all this really did make me feel special in the best kind of way. The town went and made me the grand marshal of the Christmas Parade in Savannah. It was this huge parade along the river, with floats and marching bands and fireworks . . . and elves. And me. Can you just imagine me, Ruby, being asked to be the grand marshal? That is important around here! That is something that only VIPs get asked to do. And it dawned on me that this was a big moment, not just for me, but for everyone like me. The fact that a big person could be held up high and admired—not laughed at or judged—was magical. Magical, not just because of all the twinkly lights and the fireworks overhead. But magical for me. At that moment I realized that I was helping to change the way the world sees obesity. I am making it acceptable for someone who is my size not just to go out, but to be seen, too. It was thrilling, truly. It was the best Christmas present I have ever gotten.

A Little More Than a Dozen Eyes on Me

I was just thinking today that for as many people who have come to know me on this journey, there are seven people who probably know me better than I know myself. They are Georgia, Jeff, Danna, Leslie, Marcia, Brittany, and Denny, of course. But there is someone else, too, who has a different insight, and that is my director of photography on the show, Harry Frith. He is the most incredible person ever. He has shot me and filmed me and he has seen it all. Yet he never once acted like I was fat. He sees me through the eyes of love and respect. I needed to trust him the most, and he gave me that trust. It is a wonder that people do things in their career that reflect who they truly are. When Harry looks through a camera lens, he helps us all focus on the inner truth, and I am very grateful that he has that gift.

Rosie Thoughts

I am freakin' out because someone I adore blogged about me today. You're never gonna guess who. It was Rosie O'Donnell! I swear . . . I feel so important because Rosie knows who I am and totally understands where I'm coming from. She wrote that I move her with "my grace and dignity and tiny tears." (Trust me, Rosie, they are the only thing tiny about me!) She also said my show is the only reality show that feels close to reality. What Rosie doesn't know is how many times *she* has moved me. I love her! I always have. She does such amazing things for the gay community and for kids. I have definitely learned something about being a fighter and a crusader from watching her. She says whatever's on her mind; she doesn't hold back. She speaks her thoughts because she wants good things to happen in this world. She has given a voice to so many people. You inspire me, Rosie. You really do. And if you're reading this, please know that I'd love to do something with you to support the gazillions of people—especially kids—in this nation who need help learning to love themselves just the way they are . . . whatever their struggles are. Can you imagine what two outspoken people like us could do for them together? I'd love for the chance to find out!

That's an Easy Question . . .

I am doing a lot of talking lately. People are calling me to be on their TV and radio shows and to interview me for their newspapers. I get real nervous, but I try not to show it *(sometimes if you see me twirling my hair or fiddling with my necklace, that's just me trying to contain the jitters!)*. I always try not to be too concerned with the fact that there are thousands of people watching or listening or reading (or in Oprah's case MILLIONS!). I just tell it like it is. Sometimes the questions are tough. Like when Chelsea Handler asked me, "I hear you were makin' out with Ryan Seacrest backstage?" I turned so red! I did not see that one coming! And I was *not* makin' out with Ryan (Don't I wish! He is so cute!). But I did meet him backstage and I asked him if he would ever date a big girl and he said, "Uh-huh. I would." And that just made me love him all the more. We were hugging and flirting because he is such a sweetheart!

But not all the questions I get asked are tough. An interviewer asked me one today that was very easy for me to answer. She said, "Why are you making your life so difficult? Why don't you just go and get surgery to lose the weight?" I suppose it was easy because people ask me this all the time. They want to know why am I sweating to lose all these pounds when surgery has helped so many people. Well, the answer is simple. I'm fine with other people wanting to do that, but I'm not fine with it for me.

I just want to say for the record that neither surgery nor dieting is easy no matter what. You still have to fight because you're up against a Beast. I would think about getting plastic surgery after I lose the weight because I would have so much extra skin then. It would just look all funny if I didn't. But right now, I want to lose the weight the old-fashioned way to prove to myself that *I* could do it. This is about me learning to eat right, exercise right, and get myself healthy. It's about me having the understanding and experience to keep the weight off once it comes off. Besides, I have always been scared to death of being put to sleep. Just two years ago, when I had a hernia repaired, I was *terrified*. I came through the operation fine, but I was a basket case just knowing the doctors were going to knock me out. So I told that reporter, "Look, I know I can get a quick fix; but that's not gonna help me break my addiction. That's not gonna solve anything." So I'm taking the hard road. What I mean by that is that I am searching the heart, soul, mind, physical, and spiritual part of Ruby so I can beat this addiction once and for all. It may take me longer to get where I'm going, but the bumps, the view, the stops, and the starts along this road have all been amazing—and I wouldn't trade the passengers I'm picking up along the way for anything either.

Rubyisms

I'm not quite sure when this quirky habit started, but somewhere along the way I began to create my own words. People have started calling them "Rubyisms." I think folks are beginning to know me as much for this language of mine as for my mission. One of the things someone asked me today is "What do they all mean?" Other questions I get are "Why do I use them?" and "How do I make them up?" I guess a diary is as good a place as any to confess that I really don't know.

A lot of times I have a thought or an emotion that is just too big for one word to describe. It just takes two together. My mind is a lot like the rest of me in that way—I have big ideas and big thoughts that don't fit well with some of the world's small talk, I guess. And some words just aren't nice to use around other people, though they do get to the heart of things. Most times these Rubyisms just kind of pop into my head.

The ones I'm sure I use a hundred times are just so great I forget they're not English! Some of my favorites are:

- *Natty,* which is like saying "nasty" and "bad" at the same time.
- *Nerdous,* which is like saying "nervous" and "nerdy" at the same time.
- *Humidified,* which is "humiliated" plus "horrified."
- *Uggy,* which is when something is beyond ugly.
- *Hacky* is easy—it's a combination of "happy" and "wacky."
- *Helicopter,* which is another word for where Lucifer ended up.

- *Astronaut* is my nice name for Bertha. As in, "Kiss my astronaut, y'all!"

I never realized just how addictive making up these words can be. But at least this is one addiction I don't feel the need to kick! A lot of people feel the same, and are e-mailing me their own Rubyisms. I got this one today on Facebook, and I love it so much I am gonna use it. *Exhausperated:* when you're both exhausted and exasperated. Here's another. *Hurtlarious:* when something is so darn funny, your ribs are hurting from laughing . . ." I love!

Be the Change: A Letter to President Obama

As my following grows, I feel my voice growing, too. Having so many people relying on me makes me bolder. Today I even wrote a letter to President Obama. I think it's pretty strong, too. As strong as my feelings on the subject of obesity. I think this could be the start of something major. Here's what I wrote.

> *Dear Mr. President:*
> *I have such deep respect for you, sir, that I just had to write and tell you. You are a true agent of change. And that means a lot to someone like me—someone who is trying with all my heart to make great changes in my own life and in the way others see*

people who are different. In my case, it is how others see people who are obese. You are living proof that when a person speaks the truth and takes the time to explain their thoughts, things can really take a turn for the better.

I know you are busy dealing with the recession and two wars and on top of that you are trying to do something about health care. And that's really why I am writing. I want to help be the change you are talking about, especially when it comes to health care. If you have not heard my story yet, I began at 700 pounds to educate myself about how to live a better and healthier life. I am now 333 pounds, and with every pound I have lost, I have gained new insight into this disease I call the Beast. I use the word disease because it is just that. It requires serious research, understanding, and care like any other disease. There are 72 million people fighting it in this nation right now. That is one-third of the U.S. population. And the numbers are rising. It is an epidemic. Especially among our kids.

On my journey, I have thought long and hard about how to tackle this Beast, not just for myself, but for everyone. If we don't take care of it, it will continue to take down lots of good people. I was shocked to learn that more than 85 percent of all diabetes cases are associated with obesity and being overweight; more than 70 percent of all heart-related disease is linked to being overweight and/or obese; and several kinds of cancers are heavily related to obesity and/or being overweight. I know those are a lot of numbers, and people aren't as scared of numbers as they are of reality. But that's why I am working with The Style Network to put a human face on this disease—mine. I want everyone—whether they are skinny-mini, thin, average, chunky, overweight, obese, or morbidly obese—to get what this thing is all about. But I have many more ideas than what I can fit into my show and in this letter. I would love to sit down with you to talk about ways we can make more of a difference together. Ways that won't cost the taxpayers money. Ways that can even save the taxpayers money as the levels of all these other diseases drop with the weight! I think of my TV show and my book as the best public service announcement ever, but there is so much more we can do. I know you will consider what I have to say 'cause that's what kind of person you are, so thank you in advance.

Sincerely,
Ruby Gettinger

FROM THE HEART OF CHRISTINE ACOSTA

I got to know Ruby when I moved in with my aunt and uncle, and two cousins Danna and Toni, who, at that time, lived in Savannah. I had just graduated high school. When we first met it seemed like I had known her my whole life. She has a way of making people feel that way. Ruby, Danna, Georgia, and I were pretty much inseparable. We laughed, cried, and got into all kinds of trouble. We did everything together.

One time we decided to highlight my hair, so we got one of those do-it-at-home kits. I was supposed to go out on a date that night, so I wanted to look pretty. I don't know what happened, if we left the solution on too long, or if it was just too strong for my hair, but when we were done, something just wasn't right. So we got this special shampoo that is supposed to take out brassiness. When I looked in the mirror, I was mortified (or as Ruby would say . . . humidified!). My hair was purple; it had taken on the color of the shampoo . . . I told them that they might as well just call this guy (he went to their church) and tell him not to come because I was goin' nowhere that night. Ruby kept saying, "It's not that bad . . ." She always looks on the bright side of things (though I didn't think there was such a thing as a bright side in this situation). But at least she put it into perspective: hair is hair. It's not who you are inside.

When we all grew up, we moved to different places. I went to Miami, Danna to Mississippi, Toni to South Carolina, and Ruby, for a while, to California. But through it all we were always there for each other. Sometimes in person, sometimes not. When I went through a divorce, they all came down to help me through it.

Ruby has always had an optimistic, albeit realistic, outlook on life. I know that a lot of people who get to the size that she was at her heaviest become bedridden, but I truly believe it was her love of life that kept her from that. When we would go to places like theme parks where there would be a lot of walking involved, she might have to catch her breath, or slow down now and then, but she never said, "Just go without me." She always wanted to be involved in everything. It is no surprise to me that she is where she is today—so well known and admired, inspiring people all over the country. She has always inspired me. I loves my "Rusby"!

—Christine

15   FINAL WORDS

Opening a New Door

I was so busy working on my book (and then gabbing on the phone with one of my friends for forty-five minutes) that I didn't realize how late it was getting. Time for dinner! So I went to the fridge, opened it, and began poking around inside. I was looking through this shelf and that one, pushing through some cold pizza, some of Jim's junk food, passing them over, searching for something else. There it was! The salad I made last night with grilled shrimp. Suddenly it occurred to me. I am THINKING about what I will eat. I am not just blindly pulling food out of the fridge 'cause I'm starved, trying to satisfy myself with something sweet or salty or full of fat and calories. I'm considering that protein might keep me full longer or give me energy. I am asking myself, "Have you gotten in enough fruits and veggies today?" I am controlling the food I eat, it's not controlling me. Y'all cannot believe the change in me! I am eating consciously, not just grabbing for a quick fix anymore. And it all seems so natural. I cannot wait to tell my team. It's like my brain is finally getting it. Well, today, I tell you, the Beast took a beating. There was a time when the fridge was not my friend, because it meant temptation, overindulging, and ultimately failure. It was a constant reminder of my addiction; sometimes I wish it had a big ol' chain and lock across it so I couldn't get past. But today, that was a new door I opened. Or maybe it was a new person opening it?

If God Could Change Anything . . .

I have just one more thing to add before I close this book for the night. Sometimes I wonder what I might say if God came to me tomorrow and asked, "Ruby, if you could go back in time, and I could make you fat or small . . . what would you choose?" Well, the answer just struck me and I know it to be true. I would say I'd rather be the same, Lord. I choose big. I know that sounds crazy because I am spending every second of my life fighting to get small. But I truly believe being overweight has made me a better person. It has let me sit back and observe things, see people for what they are. It has made me not take things for granted; I appreciate every little thing in life so much because of it. Really I do. I see beauty all around me because I have had to sit out on the sidelines for so long. It's a hardship, yes, but the view from those sidelines is also beauti-ful. Most people are too busy running around, never taking the time to stop, think, or feel. I do. I have. And it's because of my size that I have done this. I don't judge people; I love them unconditionally because I try to see what's beyond their shell. Walking in the shoes I've walked in has made me a bet-ter human being. So yes, God, I thank You for giving me this challenge and this gift. I don't see it as a curse like some people might. I see it as a blessing. It is good to have been where I have been, good to be where I am now, and good to be going where I know I'm headed. Plain and simple, it's good to be Ruby.

RUBY'S RESOURCE GUIDE

- Ruby's show Web site: www.mystyle.com/mystyle/shows/ruby/index.jsp
- Ourlife (formerly Hourglass): www.ourlifehealth.com
- American Diabetes Association: www.diabetes.org/home.jsp
- Brookhaven Rehabilitation Center: www.brookhavenrehab.com
- Susan G. Komen Foundation (I recently did a Breast Cancer Walk with them): ww5.komen.org/; 1.877.GO.KOMEN
- Ruby's Trainers: Drew and Shazia Edmonds, www.trainme247.com; 912-225-9695